KETTLEBELLS
for Women

KETTLEBELLS
for Women

WORKOUTS FOR YOUR STRONG, SCULPTED & SEXY BODY

Lauren Brooks

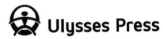 Ulysses Press

Published in the United States by
Ulysses Press
P.O. Box 3440
Berkeley, CA 94703
www.ulyssespress.com

ISBN: 978-1-61243-027-0
Library of Congress Control Number 2011934783

10 9 8 7 6 5 4 3 2

Acquisitions: Keith Riegert
Managing editor: Claire Chun
Editor: Lily Chou
Proofreader: Lauren Harrison
Production: Judith Metzener
Index: Sayre Van Young
Cover design: what!design @ whatweb.com
Cover and interior photographs: © Rapt Productions
Models: Lauren Brooks, Maya Craig, Miriam Nakamoto

Kettlebells courtesy of Dragon Door (www.dragondoor.com)

Distributed by Publishers Group West

Please Note
This book has been written and published strictly for informational purposes, and in no way should be used as a substitute for actual instruction with qualified professionals. The author and publisher are providing you with information in this work so that you can have the knowledge and can choose, at your own risk, to act on that knowledge. The author and publisher also urge all readers to be aware of their health status and to consult health care professionals before beginning any health program.

Table of Contents

PART 1

Overview

Introduction

Have you been discouraged to lift weights or do resistance training due to the fear of becoming big and bulky? Or are you just bored of the gym and not seeing the results you want? *Kettlebells for Women* is designed for any woman who wants to be strong but not bulky, who wants to lose fat without having to put in hours at the gym. This book will guide you every step of the way and explain why and how you should be using kettlebells to achieve a strong, sculpted, and sexy body in less than 30 minutes, four times a week. Thousands of women are seeing incredible results with the step-by-step programs in this book. Now it's your turn!

You may want to know that I wasn't a star athlete as a kid. I was never fully engaged in organized sports since I spent a lot of time shuttling between my father's house in Los Angeles and my mother's home in Texas. When I finally discovered surfing in high school, I tried to get into the water as much as I could.

It wasn't until I moved to California full time after high school and started surfing almost daily that I realized I wanted to focus on getting my whole body into tip-top shape. Sure, I was active enough to stop myself from getting overweight. However, I had no muscle and was far from toned. I wanted to continue to feel comfortable in a bikini while surfing, so I started working out hard and eventually developed a more muscular build. The process was so enjoyable that I decided to study kinesiology at San Diego State University. I spent my last two years of college as a personal trainer. It felt good to find my true passion.

After graduating college, I continued training clients using the tried-and-true methods to gain lean body mass and lose fat. As the years went by, however, I started losing interest in the long process it took to see results in my clients and even myself. I was sick of being indoors and seeing the machines. All I was seeing with my body was added bulk, and it wasn't helping me much with snowboarding or surfing.

Then I discovered kettlebells! They seriously changed my life. Kettlebell exercises helped freshen up stale routines and, more importantly, produced results more quickly than conventional training methods. I wanted to share the revolutionary and exciting kettlebell exercises with my clients, but the gym I was working for at the time wouldn't let me. The techniques didn't look safe and seemed dangerous. It left me no other choice. I quit and left the gym—with no clients.

I began training on my own and even flew across the country to become certified under Pavel Tsatsouline, the man responsible for popularizing kettlebells in the United States. After implementing the kettlebell methods and a new philosophy, I was more conditioned than I'd ever been in my life. My body was leaner, more sculpted, and stronger than ever. I was soon one of the first female kettlebell instructors in the San Diego area. Getting new clients wasn't difficult when people saw how effective my kettlebell training was.

Life couldn't be better—I had transformed my body, had a growing clientele, and I met the love of my life and got married. Then I became pregnant. I was overjoyed but had concerns about exercising with the kettlebells during pregnancy. Are kettlebell exercises safe for my baby? Will I lose my hard-earned six-pack? Thanks to using kettlebells safely during two pregnancies, I was clearly able to keep my strength throughout, and doctors were amazed at my quick recovery. Although I had to have two C-sections due to a breech baby, it still didn't slow me down. I owe it all to training with kettlebells and smart program design. Now it's time for you to get the same benefits as thousands of women and men who can't live without them!

A Brief History of Kettlebells

Kettlebells date back almost 300 years, although there are rumors that they could be thousands of years old, perhaps first used by Greek gladiators and athletes. The term *girya,* which means "kettlebell" in Russian, first appeared in the Russian dictionary in 1704. These heavy iron balls were used as counterweights in the markets for entertainment. Strongmen would juggle them like a circus act; the men who used these massive hunks of iron showcased unbelievable strength. As kettlebells caught on and spread in the community, they quickly became very popular. Who would've thought something so old and primitive would now be making its way into even Grandma Fay's house?

In the 1900s, the Russian community—especially athletes and bodybuilders—trained with kettlebells. Russians valued physical strength and it was quite an honor to be considered a "strongman." Kettlebells quickly became a matter of Russian national pride and a symbol of strength. A Russian strongman was referred to as a *girevik.*

In the 1980s, the Russian track and field team trained with kettlebells and won all the throwing events at the 1980 Summer Olympics in Moscow—they were unstoppable. In the military, the Russians used kettlebell exercises for their testing procedures instead of the useless push-up tests that Americans used.

In the late 1990s, Pavel Tsatsouline, a trainer for the Soviet Special Forces, became responsible for popularizing the kettlebell within the United States. You'll see and hear about kettlebells everywhere due to the incredible, rapid results most people who use this tool receive.

WHO USES THEM?

Today, unlike hundreds of years ago, kettlebells are used and enjoyed by the entire spectrum of people: men, women, boys, girls, athletes, martial artists, firefighters, Navy SEALs, celebrities, grandmas, military personnel, surgical rehab patients, and pre- and post-natal women. Because of their endless benefits and easy learning curve, kettlebells are now one of the hottest exercise tools in America. In my career as a fitness instructor, I've trained people ranging from 11-year-old kids to 85-year-old grandmothers to elite athletes. When I say kettlebells are for everyone, they really, truly are.

I have many documented success stories of people who used my kettlebell workout DVDs and achieved amazing results even though they had scoliosis, multiple sclerosis, diabetes, fibromyalgia, back pain, and more. You'll find these inspirational stories and testimonials on my blog at kbellqueen.blogspot.com and on my website at www.OnTheEdgefitness.com. If you incorporate a smart training program and effective nutrition strategies as well, you'll see great results. Make sure to check out some amazing before and after pictures on my website.

FAQ #1: *I've never done any strength training and I'm not athletic at all. Are kettlebells the right way to go?*

Kettlebell training is one of the best ways to exercise. The foundation drills contain no jarring movements and they teach the body to work together as one unit, which often prevents injury. Through the years, I've worked with many people who've either had long absences from strength training or are complete beginners. The beauty of kettlebell exercises is that they enforce proper movement patterns that carry over to all exercises and are also beneficial in everyday life. Learn the movement first and then enhance the workout by gradually adding weight. You'll be astonished with the results.

Benefits of Kettlebell Training

The benefits of kettlebell training are endless and are proving to far outshine the conventional dumbbells and fancy machines found inside gyms and health clubs. This all-around tool can actually replace almost every piece of equipment you have. The dynamic nature of the kettlebell will give you an all-in-one workout of a lifetime, combining both strength and cardio aspects.

The kettlebell's unique shape (the handle, the bulk of the weight massed into a dense ball) is obviously different than that of a dumbbell. This shape allows the body to perform a multitude of ballistic and grind exercises in a natural, fluid motion. Although most kettlebell exercises can be performed with a dumbbell, performing a snatch or a swing is much more cumbersome with a dumbbell. The dumbbell doesn't become an extension of your arm like the kettlebell since it doesn't have a handle. The kettlebell handle lets the hand hold it loosely so that the bell can float and swing outward due to the hip thrust, providing more momentum for both the upward and downward swings. With dumbbell swings, the arms are forced to be used more since the bulk of the weight is on the sides and not massed into a ball. In addition to providing incredible grip, the kettlebell handle allows for the bell to be easily passed back and forth between hands, which can keep an exercise set going for longer periods, providing an intense cardio session. The offset weight of the ball forces more muscles to stabilize and allows for the body to take each exercise through a longer range of motion. The increased range of motion will improve flexibility as well as improve the strength of deeper stabilizing muscles.

Here are some of the many benefits you'll get when using kettlebells the smart way:

- Increased endurance
- Muscular strength without the added bulk
- Full-body workout
- Rehabilitated shoulders
- Mental toughness
- Twice the results in half the time you would spend at the gym

- Rapid fat loss
- Increased core stability
- Stronger back
- Flexibility
- Decreased musculoskeletal pain

A study done by the American Council on Exercise showed the effectiveness of kettlebell training for burning calories. According to the study, doing kettlebell snatches for intervals of 15 seconds of work and 15 seconds of rest was equivalent to the calorie burn of running at a six-minute-mile pace. Since most people are unable to run that fast, this is extraordinary. The actual study had the subjects perform about 6 snatches every 15 seconds of work for 20 minutes—the calorie burn averaged out to 20.2 calories per minute! This didn't even calculate the after-burn effect on the metabolism that the body experiences after intense interval training such as this one. This quick, full-body movement proves to give the body one of the most efficient calorie-burning workouts found other than cross-country skiing.

A recent study performed in Scandinavia investigated the effects of using kettlebells to improve musculoskeletal and cardiovascular health. The study found that kettlebell training reduces pain in the neck, shoulders, and lower back. The study also showed that kettlebell training improves strength of the lower back among adults with a high prevalence of reported musculoskeletal pain.

Some of the reasons why I personally like using kettlebells:

- It decreases workout time by half.

- It saves money. No gym membership is required and you can get your entire workout done with just one bell.

- It's a full-body and very balanced workout.

- It's never boring and super fun.

- It makes your rear very strong and firm.

- It's easily transportable and can be used almost everywhere.

- It can be shared in a group setting, making it a social activity.

- It can target every single muscle group in your entire body.

- Did I say it's quick and gets to the point?

The benefits of using them are quite remarkable—it'd be silly not to implement this tool in a balanced training program.

KETTLEBELLS & PREGNANCY

I've personally had the privilege of using kettlebells throughout both of my pregnancies safely. If it weren't for training with kettlebells, my post-birth recovery wouldn't have been such a breeze. As long as you don't have any contraindications and your health-care provider allows, you, too, can continue to work with them during pregnancy.

Having short workouts to turn to during your pregnancy will make a world of difference for your mood and body. The first side effect is increased energy. Second, it relieves stress and allows the mother to be happier, which, of course, provides a safer and healthier environment for the growing baby. In addition, using kettlebells during pregnancy can, among many other positive points, help you prepare for labor by improving your strength, stamina, and mental focus; build stronger gluteal muscles (which will decrease your chances of back pain); prevent unnecessary weight gain; and accelerate post-birth recovery.

For more information on how to train safely with kettlebells during pregnancy, please check out my DVD *Baby Bells: The Fit Pregnancy Workout*, my blog at kbellqueen.blogspot.com, and my website at www.OnTheEdgefitness.com.

Before You Begin

Before you get started with the *Kettlebells for Women* program to get strong, sexy, and sculpted, there are several steps that need to be taken. As with any other program, it's very important to not jump in to it full force. That will only lead to injury and failure. To get the most out of this, you'll need to follow all of the guidelines noted here. Doing your research and educating yourself on the proper technique and taking the appropriate steps will give you long-lasting results.

DOCTOR'S PERMISSION If you have a heart condition or underlying health conditions, are pregnant, or have any physical ailments, please get your doctor's permission to perform these exercises.

PRIVATE LESSONS Many fitness enthusiasts have been quite successful learning kettlebell exercises from books, DVDs, and YouTube videos. With the growing number of professional Russian Kettlebell Challenge (RKC) certified instructors, the optimal way to learn would be to have a private lesson. If there's a certified kettlebell instructor in your area, you may want to take a lesson or two to make sure you're doing the techniques correctly. This way you can get the most out of the exercises in this book.

FOOT ATTIRE Believe it or not, the type of shoes you wear during kettlebell training can make or break it for you. Being barefoot is the ideal way to train when using kettlebells. If you're used to wearing high heels and squishy shoes, it may take you some time to get used to this, unless you do yoga or other activities while barefoot. If you've never trained barefoot, start with shoes that have flat soles. Converse, Vans, Merrell, and Vibram are all great choices for when you're outside and you feel you need to protect your feet. Tennis shoes are a bad option as they put your entire body in a posterior tilt. The heel on the shoes will also hinder your ability to root to the floor, really driving your heels in. Since your entire alignment will be off, you could injure yourself when performing many of the kettlebell drills.

ENVIRONMENT Your training environment needs to be a wide, open area with a flat, stable surface. Make sure there are no pets or kids running around you. A kettlebell can really hurt someone, so it's very important for your workout environment to be safe and open.

PROPER JUDGMENT With any exercise program, it's important to have proper judgment. If you have an injury and it hurts to lift your arm over your head, then don't do it! It's as simple as that, unless your doctor clears you to increase your range of motion. Unfortunately, I've seen people whose egos encouraged them to choose a heavier kettlebell than they were prepared for, which resulted in injury and pain. Never load bad movement patterns. Kettlebells are all about adding a challenge to already good movements. Don't let your ego get in the way. Learn to move properly, then earn the right to use the kettlebell.

Many people like to work through pain. However, pain, whether it be in your shoulder, neck, knee, hip, or back, is clearly an indicator that the body is doing something wrong and needs to be addressed immediately. For example, pressing a kettlebell over your head and feeling shoulder pain is a sign to stop or use a lighter weight. I'll never advise anyone to work through physical pain. You'll find yourself in a lot of trouble if you ignore those pain signals. To all those tough and stubborn people who like to work through pain, it's not worth it. Trust me on this one and respect your limits!

Being uncomfortable and challenging yourself safely, however, is encouraged. It's okay to work through the sensation of burning muscles as long as you don't compromise the integrity of the movement. For instance, a long set of swings might give you an uncomfortable burning in your glutes, but that's to be expected. Similarly, accelerating your heart rate and being out of breath can be uncomfortable for some. Just don't exceed your heart rate to the point of dizziness, vomiting, or fainting.

HAND PROTECTION   I've been using kettlebells for many years and have never needed gloves nor have I recommended them. Our bare hands give us immediate feedback, which helps us maneuver the kettlebell more efficiently and learn proper form. Weightlifting gloves won't allow the kettlebell to move properly in your hand. All my clients have been much better off without any weightlifting gloves.

However, just recently I discovered hand protection for those who are interested in using very heavy kettlebells. They're called New Grips and I only suggest using them for certain exercises (1- or 2-hand swings, high pulls, and renegade rows) if you choose to use a heavy bell. The majority of kettlebell users won't need this at a beginning level. If your hands get sweaty and the bell feels slippery, I suggest looking into climber's chalk—a little goes a long way. Since you don't want slippery hands, be sure not to use any kind of hand lotion prior to a kettlebell workout.

You'll develop calluses from using kettlebells frequently. The calluses are there to toughen up your hands for intense kettlebell training. The best way to keep your calluses from getting out of control is to soak them in warm water and use a pumice stone or file. Get a very good hand lotion such as Corn Huskers or use coconut oil. You can still have nice hands, but don't be afraid of small calluses. Like I always say, "Nice hands or a nice ass?"

WRIST AND FOREARM PROTECTION   If you have sensitive wrists, you may want to look into getting wrist bands. Any cushy sweat band will do. These will just provide protection for the area around the wrist and forearm when learning some of the kettlebell moves or getting used to having the bell rest on that area. Most of my clients don't use wrist protection, but I prefer people use them rather than having bruises from bad form. Learn the form properly so you don't need them, but if you're sensitive, please use wrist bands to make kettlebells fun for you.

Nutrition for Optimal Health & Fat Loss

"Let food be thy medicine and medicine be thy food."
—Hippocrates

Many people who work out daily still battle weight and health problems. Having a well-designed workout plan will definitely help you get stronger and leaner as well as burn fat. However, without focusing on proper nutrition, getting optimal results will be extremely hard and not possible for most people. Frequently athletes, marathon runners, and exercise fanatics come to me for nutrition advice. They complain about how hard they work out and wonder why they never lose a pound and their clothes always fit the same. As soon as we start cleaning up their diet, immediately the pounds start coming off and their energy skyrockets. In fact, many times they even cut back on exercise and still lose weight just from eating better.

One problem with frequent exercisers is that they feel they earned a treat or worked for their pizza and beer. Remember: The calories that you burn during exercise can be replaced in less than five minutes. If you're one of those people who think just exercising alone, without making significant dietary changes, is going to shed the pounds, then you're truly fooling yourself.

For the purposes of this book, this nutrition section will only serve as a guide. Rather than define what a macronutrient or a calorie is, I'll just get to the point: To build a healthy, functioning body that'll last, proper nutrition must be the number-one priority. I'm not talking about calorie counting, point systems, or obsessing over macronutrient percentages, since always having to be a mathematician with your food is just not a realistic lifestyle that the majority of us can sustain. Focusing on real foods that are nutrient rich will be the absolute best way to not only fuel your body for optimal health, but to get you to the weight and lean body that you were meant to have.

Knowing what, when, and how to fuel your body will be very important in achieving your goals. Without a doubt, getting your nutrition from whole foods that are in their most natural state should be number one on your list. The more the food has been changed, processed, heated, or pre-cut, the more the nutrient value diminishes. Fresh, raw vegetables and seasonal organic fruits should make up the bulk of your diet. Protein from organic, free-range, properly fed animals, legumes, raw nuts and seeds, and whole grains should also be part of a healthy diet. Vegetarians and vegans who eat a healthy, high plant-based diet have proven that the ample protein and nutrition from plant sources allow them to maintain their strength.

Avoid foods that are processed with refined sugars, including bagels, muffins, and most packaged cereals and bars. Fake meats, deli meat, and overly pasteurized dairy products filled with hormones should also be avoided.

Everyone has different lifestyles and metabolisms, therefore telling everyone that they need to eat every two to three hours is not always the best way to go. With my experience designing hundreds of personalized nutrition programs, I've found that most people do well eating every two to four hours. It sustains them and keeps them from overeating due to the starving sensation. However, a select group can succeed using the "Warrior Diet" method. This method involves grazing on very little food throughout the day to keep energy levels up, then eating the main meal in the evening. I personally like a happy medium (i.e., not stuffing myself during the day to avoid the post-lunch crash).

The following are sample meal plans for omnivores and strict vegetarians.

BREAKFAST

Meaty option

16 oz water (2 8-oz glasses) upon waking

1 veggie omelet or scramble; use 3 organic free-range eggs (1 yolk and 2 whites), 1 cup fresh arugula or spinach, and any vegetables you desire

Small bowl of berries

Vegetarian option

16 oz water (2 8-oz glasses) upon waking

⅓ cup organic oatmeal

1 Tbs chia seeds

1 serving blueberries

MID-MORNING

Option 1

1 apple or pear

2 Tbs organic peanut or almond butter

Option 2

8–12 oz fresh-squeezed green juice with kale, cucumber, parsley, apple, lemon, and ginger

LUNCH

Meaty option

2 cups organic greens (e.g., baby spinach, arugula) topped with cucumbers, tomatoes, green onions

1–2 Tbs light dressing

3–4 oz wild river fish or organic free-range chicken or turkey

1 small yam

Vegetarian option

Make same salad but replace meat with 1 serving hummus, beans, or lentils

AFTERNOON or PRE-/POST-WORKOUT SNACK

Option 1

Organic nonfat plain Greek yogurt

Handful crushed walnuts

½ cup organic blueberries

1 tsp agave or yacon syrup

Option 2

Pre- or Post-Workout Smoothie:

Raw, organic, sprouted brown rice protein

8 oz unsweetened almond milk

Banana

1 Tbs chia seeds

DINNER

Meaty option

3–4 oz organic chicken breast or grass-fed beef

10 asparagus spears, lightly grilled

½ cup butternut squash

Vegetarian option

Fist-size portion cooked quinoa

Large veggie stir-fry with broccolini, garlic, onions, asparagus

Handful cashews with splash of lime juice stirred in

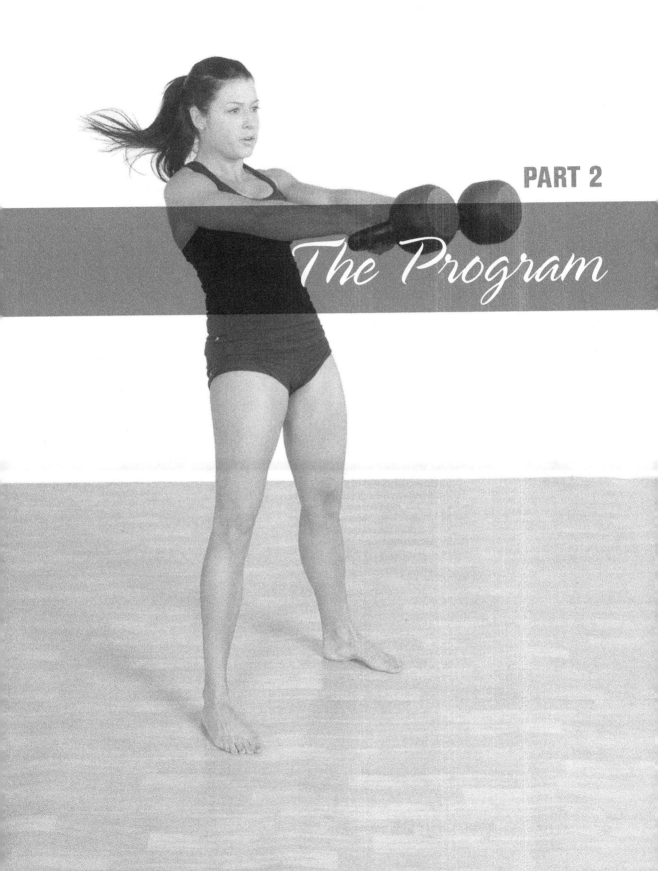

PART 2

The Program

How to Use This Book

This book is a great resource for anyone who wants a large variety of exercises to choose from as well as different-level workouts to follow. But before you jump into the *Kettlebells for Women* program (page 21), make sure to read through the safety section (page 12) and browse through the exercises in Part 3. The nutrition section (page 14) will be an important component if you want to achieve fat loss along with body sculpting and an energy boost.

If you've been using kettlebell workout DVDs at home and feel like you're missing important instruction, chances are the exercise is detailed in this book. Spend some time reading the detailed instructions in Part 3, practice the movements daily, and your follow-along workout session will soon be a breeze. This in turn will allow you to move with confidence, have better form, and amplify your fat-loss, strengthening, and sculpting goals.

If you prefer making your own programs, pick one or two exercises from every section and create your own balanced workouts. You can mix and match to the point where you can have a new workout daily. No matter how you use this book, have fun!

CHOOSING YOUR KETTLEBELL

Generally our bodies can lift and swing much heavier than we can press. Therefore, lighter bells are used more for upper-body exercises (e.g., overhead lifts, get-ups, windmills) while heavier bells are used for lower-body exercises (e.g., deadlifts, swings). In a perfect world, you'd have several sizes on hand to choose from. As you get stronger and more skilled, you'll want to increase the size of the kettlebell you use.

Here are my suggestions for kettlebell package purchases for both single- and double-kettlebell exercises.

	Single-Kettlebell Exercises	*Double-Kettlebell Exercises*
Beginner	6kg, 8kg, and 12kg (13lb, 18lb, and 25lb)	pair of 6kg or 8kg (13lb or 18lb)
Intermediate	8kg, 12kg, and 16kg (18lb, 25lb, and 35lb)	pair of 8kg or 12kg (18lb or 25lb)
Advanced (Very Strong)	12kg, 16kg, 20kg, and 24kg (25lb, 35lb, 44lb, and 53lb)	pair of 12kg or/and 16kg (25lb or/and 35lb)

High-quality kettlebells can be pricey so don't be discouraged if you can only afford one right now. Here are my recommendations for each level.

> **Fragile:** 4kg (9lb) or 6kg (13lb)
> **Average:** 8kg (18lb)
> **Strong:** 12kg (25lb)
> **Very strong:** 16kg (35lb)

Keep in mind that these are just suggestions, not requirements. If you already have dumbbells or some cheaper small bells, you can use those in exercises that suggest a lighter bell or no bell, such as the Turkish get-up, windmills, and presses. When I first started out I only had one 8kg (18lb) Dragon Door kettlebell. Then my collection turned to two when I added a 12kg/25lb. Now I have, well, too many to count!

FAQ #3: *I stopped lifting weights because I develop muscle easily. Will kettlebells make me bulky?*

When working all the muscle groups at once, the body will get strong but still look trim and lean. If you've never done any strength training, naturally a small amount of muscle growth may occur, but nothing that will result in a bulky look. The muscle will be useful and strong, as well as help to increase your metabolism for extra fat burning. Some of my smallest, leanest female clients are working with super-heavy kettlebells that they'd never have thought possible. An article I wrote on this subject has been translated into several languages. You can read it on my website at www.OnTheEdgeFitness.com. Now go get strong!

Most beginners are concerned that they'll move up quickly in size and that buying lighter kettlebells will be a waste of money. However, even my strongest clients reach for light kettlebells for joint mobility, warm-ups, and advanced moves such as bottoms-up presses. Trust me: Your light kettlebell will get plenty of use. They'll be good for active recovery and days when you just want to have an easy day or learn a new technique.

Styles & Brands

There are many different styles and brands of kettlebells to choose from. I began my training with kettlebells made by the company that Pavel Tsatsouline, the kettlebell king himself, partnered up with: Dragon Door. These bells are the Cadillac of all kettlebells. Their design ensures proper wrist alignment; their texture prevents you from ripping your hands. I've test-driven quite a few bells and these are still number one in my book. A few cheaper brands are also acceptable and will definitely work. You can read my reviews under the FAQ section on my website www.OnTheEdgeFitness.com.

WARMING UP & COOLING DOWN

Warming up should be a part of every workout that you do. Warming up properly can help prevent injury, make sure that the right muscles are fired up and activated, and allow you to ease into your workouts safely. Some of the warm-up drills will feel like easier versions of the actual workouts, but going through the motions should allow your body to loosen up and help create better blood flow for the entire workout. Think of these as pre-exercises for better performance. In the workout programs, I've included days for just joint mobility and warm-up drills. Take 5–10 minutes out of your day to perform these exercises.

Moving around at a slower place, whether walking slowly or slowing down intense movement, is the best way to gradually lower your heart rate to its resting rate. Abruptly stopping after an intense training without cooling down can be problematic—you might become dizzy and faint. You might also experience blood pooling, which occurs when the heart rate suddenly drops from insufficient cool-down, causing the veins to shrink. The result: The build-up of blood has a difficult time pumping back to the heart effectively.

Stretches are best done after you've worked out and cooled down slightly but still have warm muscles. The purpose of stretching is to increase flexibility and range of motion. Choose the stretches that you feel your body needs and make sure to stretch both sides. Inhale deeply through your nose and breathe all your air out as you continue your stretch. Relaxed breathing is optimal during all stretches. If you'd like to further your stretching, I recommend Pavel Tsatsouline's book *Relax into Stretch*. It offers great techniques on how to really unlock and develop flexibility with his proven stretching method.

Joint mobility is key for range of motion and relieving stiffness. Every time you perform a rep, you allow synovial fluid to "oil" each joint for better movement; stretching alone won't do this. Having lubricated joints will make all the difference in your training and as you age. Think of it as anti-aging medicine for your body. Doing joint mobility for warm-up and cool-down can prevent injury. In fact, stretching still hasn't been proven to prevent injury. You're better off with joint mobility if you have to pick between the two.

REST & ACTIVE RECOVERY

One of the first questions I get from a new client or someone enthusiastic about kettlebell training is how often she can work out with kettlebells. The answer is: It all depends. There are many variables (e.g., intensity, program design, goals, outside stressors, fitness level, proper technique) that go along with the optimal frequency of kettlebell use. Do some people use kettlebells every day? Sure. Do I recommend this to everyone? Absolutely not. Each person has a different response to exercise and proper recovery is very important to not only avoid injury and burnout but to succeed.

Many exercise fanatics or people who dive in headfirst don't realize that not taking proper rest will actually hinder their progress. If you don't allow your body to recover, you'll not only burn out, you may regress in your training, meaning you won't see improvements and gains. Training too hard can lead to overtraining and the frying of the central nervous system. Hard exercise is a stressor on the body that releases stress hormones. Make sure you take your recovery and rest time seriously so that you can continue this journey for a lifetime.

Active rest/recovery using light exercises (such as walking, light biking, easy yoga, joint mobility, stretching, and light swings), rather than just plain resting, has recently been shown to produce positive effects after or during a hard workout. They'll all keep your body mobile and assist in the recovery process. All in all, incorporating active rest after a hard workout or between workouts will allow you to come back stronger. More and more professional athletes are using active recovery as a method to enhance their performance. There's no reason why everyone shouldn't implement active recovery in their own program.

The Ultimate Strong, Sexy, and Sculpted Kettlebell Program

This carefully designed 12-week program includes 15 different workouts for people of all fitness levels. It also includes three bonus Tabata workouts, which are metabolic boosters. The beauty of this comprehensive program is that it allows you to explore new options for constantly improving and changing your body, whether using heavier weights or incorporating different exercise choices. This program will not only sculpt and tone your entire body, but help you become very strong and conditioned without the added bulk. What woman doesn't want to be strong, sexy, and sculpted using a no-nonsense, time-saving approach?

If you're an exercise enthusiast, you don't have to give up your other activities, whether they be running, walking, yoga, swimming, cycling, martial arts, tennis, or surfing. You can still do all of your favorite activities along with kettlebells. If you practice yoga three times a week and begin implementing kettlebells into your program, I recommend doing yoga on your "Active Recovery/Joint Mobility" days. If you like to walk, you can still walk every day. If you're a runner, when first beginning kettlebell training, add your runs on your "off" kettlebell days. Unless you're training for a competition, the most important thing is to find that perfect balance for yourself.

Before you begin, make sure to read "Choosing Your Kettlebell" (page 18) carefully in order to help you select the appropriate kettlebell for your level and exercise. The strength gains and body fat loss will come nicely with a slow, safe progression. Those who aren't patient and don't pace themselves generally end up burning out. Slow and steady will win the race with this one. Spend the extra time on form and technique. Listen very closely to your body, use common sense, and you'll see the incredible results that you worked hard for.

USING THE PROGRAM

There are three levels in this program. The first four weeks of the program are all about building the foundation for success. Beginners will need to start here to learn basics such as the deadlift, swing, clean, press, and squat. If you're unsure of your form or have limitations, make sure to get a kettlebell lesson in person from a local certified kettlebell instructor. If it hurts, you're probably doing it wrong. This applies to all levels! Once you complete Level 1 and have that strong foundation, you'll be ready for the more demanding workouts in the program. If you feel that you're not ready to progress to the more challenging weeks or levels in this program, your body will thank you for spending the extra time repeating the same section. Building your structural integrity is the most important part now. Don't be fooled with the simplicity of this design.

If you've been using kettlebells on your own for more than a year and feel that you have perfect form and technique, you may start with Level 2. However, since you can never practice the foundational exercises enough, my recommendation is for everyone to start at the beginning. Even advanced athletes spend ample time refining their basic form for optimal gains in strength and injury prevention. If something is too easy, swap it for a more advanced option (noted either in the workout itself or in the Part 3 exercise description). Other options include using heavier bells, increasing reps, adding speed, and resting less.

No matter what your fitness level, make sure to spend a good 5, 10, or even 15 minutes on the warm-up and/or joint mobility exercises (see pages 125–47) before beginning these workouts. For increased flexibility and range of motion, perform joint mobility and stretching in the cool-down period, after you complete the workout.

After completing the entire program once, you can start it again, but this time using a heavier kettlebell or/and choosing some of the more-advanced exercises for the assigned workout of the day. Everything else in life will feel easier once you get through this program. Take advantage of all the exercises to cycle back and start the program again with heavier weights and/or more advanced exercises.

As you become a seasoned kettlebell user, you'll learn how to create your own programs. For example, if a workout calls for Double Squats, you can substitute them with Single-Leg Squats for more of a challenge. If a workout calls for the Single-Bell Military Press, you can make it harder by choosing the Double Press or the Seesaw Press. Feel free to get creative and add in some variety, but only after you've really mastered the standard exercises.

KEY TERMS

Here are terms and concepts you'll want to familiarize yourself with in order to get the most out of this program.

Reps The number of repetitions called for each particular exercise. If you see 15 reps of swings, you'll perform 15 swings with no rest in between.

Sets The number of times you perform each exercise. For example, 10 squats and 10 swings for 3 sets means you'll perform each exercise 10 times and then repeat for a total of 3 different times. This could be done with or without rest between each set, depending on the type of workout.

Failure The physical state when you can no longer complete another repetition. Training to failure can be very dangerous not only for your muscles but for your central nervous system; it can actually cause your body to regress. Only practice perfect reps and stop a movement when you know that you won't be able to perform the next rep with proper form or can't complete it at all. Your body will learn incorrect movement patterns when you force it to complete a rep that it may not be capable of doing. For the timed workouts in this program, make sure to stop early if you know you're doing it wrong. This will be paramount in making progress and not regressing or burning out.

Intensity The effort you put toward each exercise within the workout. This will be an important aspect of your training to understand. One of the reasons why people get such great results when using kettlebells is because of the intensity they can bring to each session. Kettlebell swings are supposed to be done with a high amount of intensity. Even if you use a light kettlebell, you still need to swing that bell with strong, ballistic intent.

Not every workout will be extremely challenging, though. Varying intensity is important for your body and mind. In general, you should give each workout your all, keeping it intense but safe. However, intensity doesn't give you the green light to take your exercise to failure or perform a movement with bad form. Because I expect everyone to work out with a higher intensity, naturally the workouts will be for a shorter duration, otherwise the intensity level will drop since people lose intensity with longer, more endurance-type workouts. For the purpose of the program in this book, shorter, more-intense sessions done more frequently will give you the most bang for your buck. You'll also leave these workouts not feeling drained and will have more energy than you did prior to starting the workout.

Power breath   The way of breathing that braces your core to protect your back and give you more power throughout your exercise. You'll find that I refer to the power breath in many of the exercise instructions. There are two different types of breathing used in kettlebell training: slow (slow tension breathing) and quick (power breathing). Pavel Tsatsouline borrows the phrase "breathing behind the shield" from *Uechi-ryu* karate practitioners. To perform slow tension breath, make the "s" sound and hiss for a few seconds, like air leaking out of a tire. While you're hissing, feel your stomach and see how it braces. This is an important breathing technique to utilize during slower exercises such as presses, single-leg deadlifts, and squats. To perform power breathing, exhale quickly and sharply with either a "huh" or "s" sound. This is a perfect bracing mechanism for fast, ballistic exercises like swings, cleans, and snatches.

Tension   Tension is strength, so to speak. Developing tension throughout your body will allow you to lift heavier weights. If I squeeze all my muscles together by tensing each one from head to toe while pressing up a heavy kettlebell, I'll have more tension to allow the lift to be completed. Even making a fist will create more blood flow for increased strength. For example, if you're going to push a car, you'll naturally have the most success by grounding your lower body to the pavement, leaning into the car with tense arms, and pushing with all your might. If you were relaxed and none of your muscles were tensing, you wouldn't have much luck. The same thing applies to lifting weights. You'll find yourself moving heavier weights by squeezing the appropriate muscles for that particular exercise. However, constantly creating tension will cause you to tire out more quickly. Be sure to use tension techniques only when you have to, otherwise you won't be able to last very long.

Sequence   The order in which exercises should be performed. Some workouts include several sequences. In these scenarios, complete a full sequence of exercises in the order listed for the suggested reps and sets, then start the following sequence of exercises.

Tabata   The Tabata method was started by Dr. Izumi Tabata in the mid-1990s at the National Institute of Fitness and Sports in Tokyo, Japan. Tabata's team discovered after using various intense protocols that 8 rounds of 20 seconds of all-out max effort followed by 10 seconds of rest for a total 4 minutes produced extraordinary measurable results. Improvements such as fat loss, aerobic conditioning, athletic performance, and anaerobic threshold were shown. I personally love Tabata interval training since it's efficient and delivers amazing results. That's why I've included bonus Tabata workouts.

INTERVAL TRAINING

Interval training, or working for a predetermined amount of time or number of reps then taking a short break before continuing, has been shown to be very effective. It allows you to make each exercise much more challenging. For example, you could do an interval circuit of push-ups, swings, and squats by performing each exercise for 15 seconds for as fast as you can, then taking a 15-second rest before moving on to the next exercise. By raising the intensity, you'll not only burn more calories throughout the workout, you'll get the afterburn for the next 24–48 hours. Get in the habit of incorporating more interval training into your life—you'll notice much quicker fat-burning results overall.

LEVEL ONE: KETTLEBELL FOUNDATION AND FAT LOSS

Month 1 (Weeks 1–4)

	Week 1	Week 2	Week 3	Week 4
Monday	Workout 1	Rest	Workout 4	Rest
Tuesday	Joint Mobility/ Active Recovery	Workout 3	Joint Mobility/ Active Recovery	Workout 4
Wednesday	Workout 2	Workout 2	Workout 5	Joint Mobility + Tabata 1
Thursday	Joint Mobility/ Active Recovery	Joint Mobility/ Active Recovery	Rest	Workout 5
Friday	Workout 1	Workout 3	Workout 3	Joint Mobility/ Active Recovery
Saturday	Rest	Joint Mobility/ Active Recovery	Joint Mobility + Tabata 1	Workout 4
Sunday	Workout 2	Rest	Workout 2	Workout 1 + Tabata 1

Everyone progresses at different levels. If you're not ready to start Month 2, spend a few more weeks to a month at Level 1.

LEVEL ONE WARM-UP Use this warm-up before starting any of the Level 1 workouts. If you have extra time, feel free to add any joint mobility exercise (pages 138–47) to this warm-up.

Exercise	Time/Reps	Comments
Floor Bridge *p. 126*	8 reps	
Hip Opener & Glute Activator *p. 128*	8 reps each side	
Ankle Mobility *p. 129*	5 reps each side	
Kneeling Halo *p. 131*	8 reps each direction	lightest bell you have
Hip Hinge *p. 41*	8 reps	
Bodyweight Squat *p. 132*	5 reps	use your elbows to gently pry your knees open at the bottom
Lateral Lunge *p. 133*	3 reps each side	

WORKOUT 1 Go through each exercise and perform the suggested reps. Take a short rest if needed between each exercise. Repeat the entire sequence for a total of 2–3 sets.

Start with Level One Warm-Up (page 24).		
Exercise	**Reps**	**Rest**
Deadlift p. 42	10	0–30 sec
1-Arm Swing p. 50	5 each arm	0–30 sec
Chest Press p. 84	5	0–30 sec
Suitcase Deadlift p. 43	5 each arm	0–30 sec
2-Arm Swing p. 49	10	0–30 sec
Repeat this sequence a total of 2–3 times.		

WORKOUT 2 Perform the suggested reps for each exercise, moving on to the next after a brief rest. After you complete all the exercises, rest for 30–60 seconds and start again with the first exercise listed.

Start with Level One Warm-Up (page 24).		
Exercise	**Reps**	**Rest**
Goblet Squat p. 105	5	brief
Single-Arm Row p. 90	8	brief
Deadlift p. 42	8	brief
Clean p. 55	5 each arm	brief
1-Arm Swing p. 50	6 each arm	30–60 sec
If this is your first week, only perform this workout 1 or 2 times. If this is week 3 or 4, you may perform this workout 2 to 3 times.		

WORKOUT 3   This is a timed workout, so set your timer for 30 seconds. Perform an exercise for 30 seconds, rest for 30 seconds, then move on to the next exercise.

Start with Level One Warm-Up (page 24).		
Exercise	*Time*	*Rest*
Beg: Squat p. 104 **Int/Adv:** Goblet Squat p. 105	30 sec	30 sec
Beg: Clean p. 55 and Military Press p. 60 **Int:** Double Clean p. 56 and Double Military Press p. 60	30 sec	30 sec
2-Arm Swing p. 49	30 sec	30 sec
1-Arm Plank Hold p. 88 (Alternate back and forth, holding each side for 2 seconds. Work your way up to 10 reps total.)	30 sec	30 sec
Alternating Swing p. 52	30 sec	30 sec
Waiter Walk (1 bell) p. 68	30 sec each side	30 sec
Repeat for a total of 3–4 sets, depending on your fitness level.		

WORKOUT 4   This is a timed workout, so set your timer for 30 seconds. Perform an exercise for 30 seconds, rest for 30 seconds, then move on to the next exercise.

Start with Level One Warm-Up (page 24).		
Exercise	*Time*	*Rest*
Beg: Deadlift p. 42 **Int/Adv:** Deadlift (2 bells) p. 42	30 sec	30 sec
Clean (left) p. 55	30 sec	30 sec
Clean (right) p. 55	30 sec	30 sec
Bodyweight Push-Up p. 75	30 sec	30 sec
2-Arm Swing p. 49	30 sec	30 sec
Repeat for a total of 3–4 sets, depending on your fitness level.		

WORKOUT 5   Perform this workout with a brief rest in between each exercise.

Exercise	Reps	Rest
Start with Level One Warm-Up (page 24).		
Sequence A		
Beg: Half-Kneeling Press (less strong side) *p. 67* **Int/Adv:** Clean *p. 55* and Military Press *p. 60* (less strong side) or Half Kneeling Press, *p. 67*	5	brief
Beg: Half-Kneeling Press (stronger side) *p. 67* **Int/Adv:** Clean *p. 55* and Military Press *p. 60*	5	brief
Beg: Stationary Lunge *p. 109* **Int/Adv:** Stationary Lunge with Bell *p. 110*	5 each side	30–60 sec
Repeat for a total of 2–3 sets. Rest as needed before starting Sequence B.		
Sequence B		
1-Arm Swing *p. 50*	10 each side	30 sec
High Plank *p. 136*	30 sec	30 sec
2-Arm Swing *p. 49*	20	30–60 sec
Repeat for a total of 2–3 sets.		

TABATA 1   This is a bonus metabolic conditioning workout that lasts 4 minutes. Repeat 4 rounds total.

Exercise	Time	Sets	Rest
2-Arm Swing *p. 49*	20 sec	4	10 sec
Squat Thrust *p. 134*	20 sec	4	10 sec

LEVEL TWO: STRENGTH AND FAT BURNING
Month 2 (Weeks 5–8)

	Week 5	Week 6	Week 7	Week 8
Monday	Joint Mobility + Tabata 2	Workout 8	Workout 7	Rest
Tuesday	Workout 6	Rest	Joint Mobility/ Active Recovery	Workout 6
Wednesday	Joint Mobility/ Active Recovery	Joint Mobility + Tabata 2	Workout 10	Joint Mobility + Tabata 2
Thursday	Workout 7	Workout 9	Joint Mobility/ Tabata 2	Workout 9
Friday	Rest	Joint Mobility/ Active Recovery	Workout 8	Joint Mobility/ Active Recovery
Saturday	Workout 8	Workout 6	Rest	Workout 10
Sunday	Joint Mobility + Tabata 2	Rest	Workout 9	Joint Mobility + Tabata 2

LEVEL TWO WARM-UP Use this warm-up before starting any of the Level Two workouts.

Exercise	Time/Reps	Comments
Floor Bridge p. 126	5 reps	
Single-Leg Floor Bridge p. 127	8 reps each side	
Ankle Mobility p. 29	5 reps each side	
Kneeling Halo p. 131	8 reps each direction	lightest bell you have
Mini Plank p. 125	8 reps	rest 6 sec and repeat 6 times
Bodyweight Squat p. 132	5 reps	use your elbows to gently pry your knees open at the bottom
Lateral Lunge p. 133	5 reps each side	
Farmer's Walk p. 133	20 sec each side	

WORKOUT 6   Follow the specific directions for each sequence. Once you complete the first sequence for the suggested sets, rest 1–2 minutes, or as needed, and begin Sequence B feeling fresh.

Start with Level Two Warm-Up (page 28).		
Exercise	**Reps**	**Rest**
Sequence A Set your timer for 30 seconds. Perform an exercise for 30 seconds, rest for 30 seconds, then move on to the next exercise.		
Beg: Chest Press p. 84 **Int:** 1-Arm Floor Press (left/right) p. 85 **Adv:** Seesaw Floor Press p. 86	30 sec	30 sec
Clean p. 55 and Front Squat (left) p. 105	30 sec	30 sec
Clean p. 55 and Front Squat (right) p. 105	30 sec	30 sec
Beg: Alternating Swing p. 52 **Int/Adv:** Double Swing p. 53	30 sec	1–3 min
Repeat 2–4 rounds, depending on your fitness level. Rest as needed before starting Sequence B.		
Sequence B Set your timer for 20 seconds. Perform as many perfect reps of each exercise as you can in 20 seconds. Take a 20-second break and move on to the next exercise.		
Pullover to Crunch p. 97	20 sec	20 sec
Russian Twist p. 100	20 sec	20 sec
Mini Plank p. 125	20 sec	20 sec
Farmer's Walk (2 bells) p. 133	20 sec	20 sec
Rest then repeat 2–4 rounds.		

WORKOUT 7   Perform the Sequence A exercises one after the other with little rest in between. Once 2–3 rounds are completed, move on to Sequence B. Rest before performing Sequence C.

Start with Level Two Warm-Up (page 28).		
Exercise	**Reps**	**Rest**
Sequence A		
Beg: Bodyweight Windmill, *p. 70* **Int:** Windmill (Bottom) *p. 71* **Adv:** Windmill (Top) *p. 72*	3 each side	minimal
Beg: Single-Leg Deadlift *p. 46* **Int:** Single-Leg Deadlift (1 bell) *p. 46* **Adv:** Single-Leg Deadlift (2 bells) *p. 46*	6 each side	minimal
Hand-to-Hand Swing *p. 52*	12	minimal
Rest then repeat 2 rounds. Rest as needed before starting Sequence B.		
Sequence B Set timer for 20 seconds on, 20 seconds off.		
Deck Squat *p. 108*	20 sec	20 sec
Beg: Push-Up on Knees *p. 75* (bells optional) *p. 76* **Int/Adv:** Push-Up *p. 75* (bells optional) *p. 77*	20 sec	20 sec
Single-Arm Row (right) *p. 90*	20 sec	20 sec
Single-Arm Row (left) *p. 90*	20 sec	20 sec
High Pull (right) *p. 115*	20 sec	20 sec
High Pull (left) *p. 115*	20 sec	20 sec
Rest as needed before starting Sequence C.		
Sequence C Repeat for 2–3 rounds.		
Russian Twist *p. 100*	20 sec	20 sec
Mini Plank *p. 125*	20 sec	20 sec

WORKOUT 8 Go through each sequence and perform the suggested reps and sets. Rest 30–60 seconds if needed before moving on to the next sequence. Feel free to practice joint mobility or hip flexor stretches in between each sequence.

Start with Level Two Warm-Up (page 28).		
Exercise	**Reps**	**Rest**
Sequence A		
Get-Up Sit-Up p. 118	1 each side	minimal
Turkish Get-Up (with or without weight) p. 119	1 each side	30–60 sec
Repeat 3 times. Rest as needed before starting Sequence B.		
Sequence B		
Bottoms-Up Clean (light bell) p. 59	3 each side	minimal
Goblet Squat p. 105	5–8	minimal
2-Arm Swing p. 49	20	30–60 sec
Repeat 2 times. Rest as needed before starting Sequence C.		
Sequence C		
Tall Kneeling Press p. 66 or Seated Press p. 65	5 each side	minimal
Biceps Curl p. 95	8–10	minimal
Triceps Extension p. 94	8	minimal
Snatch p. 123	5 each side	30–60 sec
Repeat 2 times.		

WORKOUT 9 Perform the Sequence A exercises for the suggested amount of reps, resting 30 seconds between each exercise.

Start with Level Two Warm-Up (page 28).		
Sequence A		
Exercise	**Reps**	**Rest**
Beg: Double-Bell Push-Up *p. 77* **Int/Adv:** Single-Bell Diamond Push-Up *p. 78*	5–8	30 sec
Beg: Single-Leg Squat on Bench *p. 107* **Int/Adv:** Forward Lunge *p. 112*	5 each side	30 sec
Beg: Double Suitcase Deadlift *p. 44* **Int/Adv:** Sumo Deadlift (2 bells) *p. 45*	5	30 sec
Beg: 2-Arm Swing *p. 49* **Int/Adv:** Double Swing *p. 53*	15	30–60 sec
Repeat 3–4 times. Rest as needed before starting Sequence B.		
Sequence B		
Pullover *p. 96*	30 sec	30 sec
Russian Twist *p. 100*	30 sec	30 sec
Side Plank (left) *p. 99*	30 sec	30 sec
Side Plank (right) *p. 99*	30 sec	30 sec
Repeat for a total of 2–3 rounds.		

WORKOUT 10 Perform the exercises in each sequence one after the next for the suggested reps. Repeat each sequence 2–3 rounds before moving on to the next sequence. Rest 1–3 minutes between each sequence.

Start with Level Two Warm-Up (page 28).		
Exercise	**Reps**	**Rest**
Sequence A		
Turkish Get-Up p. 119	3 each side	minimal
1-Arm Swing p. 50	8 each side	minimal
Repeat 2–3 rounds. Rest 1–3 minutes as needed before starting Sequence B.		
Sequence B		
Beg: Renegade Row p. 89 **Int:** Stabilized Plank Single-Arm Row, p. 91	Alternate 4 each side	minimal
Kickstand Lunge p. 114	8 each side	minimal
Push Press p. 64	8 each side	minimal
High Pull p. 115	8 each side	minimal
Repeat 2–3 rounds. Rest 1–3 minutes before starting Sequence C.		
Sequence C		
Janda Sit-Up p. 98	30 sec	minimal
Side Plank p. 99	30 sec each side	minimal
Renegade Hold p. 58	15 sec each side	30–60 sec
Rest 30–60 seconds. Repeat 2–3 rounds.		

TABATA 2 This is a bonus metabolic conditioning workout. Go through all the exercises for 20 seconds of all-out work and 10 seconds of rest. Start at the top and repeat for a total of 2 sets. If you're more advanced, take a 1-minute break after the 2 sets and repeat the entire section again for another 2 sets.

Exercise	**Time**	**Sets**	**Rest**
1-Arm Swing (left) p. 50	20 sec	2	10 sec
2-Arm Swing (right) p. 49	20 sec	2	10 sec
Squat Thrust p. 134	20 sec	2	10 sec
Jumping Jacks p. 136	20 sec	2	10 sec

LEVEL THREE: POWERHOUSE STRENGTH AND CONDITIONING
Month 3 (Week 9–12)

	Week 9	Week 10	Week 11	Week 12
Monday	Workout 11	Joint Mobility/ Active Recovery	Workout 14	Rest
Tuesday	Rest	Workout 13	Joint Mobility/ Active Recovery	Workout 12
Wednesday	Joint Mobility + Tabata 3	Rest	Workout 15	Joint Mobility/ Active Recovery
Thursday	Workout 12	Workout 14	Joint Mobility + Tabata 3	Workout 14
Friday	Joint Mobility + Tabata 3	Joint Mobility + Tabata 3	Workout 12	Joint Mobility/ Active Recovery
Saturday	Rest	Workout 13	Rest	Workout 15
Sunday	Workout 2	Rest	Workout 2	Joint Mobility + Tabata 3

LEVEL THREE WARM-UP   Use this warm-up before starting any of the Level Three workouts.

Exercise	Time/Reps	Comments
Floor Bridge p. 126	5 reps	
Single-Leg Floor Bridge p. 127	8 reps each side	
Ankle Mobility p. 129	5 reps each side	
Halo p. 130	8 reps each direction	lightest bell you have
Mini Plank p. 125	10 sec	rest 10 sec and repeat 4 times
Bodyweight Squat p. 132	10 reps	use your elbows to gently pry your knees open at the bottom
Rack Walk p. 58	30 sec each arm	
Lateral Lunge p. 133	5 reps each side	
Farmer's Walk (2 bells) p. 133	30 sec	

WORKOUT 11 Perform the Sequence A exercises one after the next for 3 rounds. Sequence B is a complex, so don't set the bells down until you complete the third exercise in the sequence.

Start with Level Three Warm-Up (page 34).		
Exercise	**Reps**	**Rest**
Sequence A		
Single-Leg Squat on Bench p. 107	5 each side	none
Double Swing p. 53	10	none
Repeat 3 times. Rest 1–3 minutes as needed before starting Sequence B.		
Sequence B Perform each exercise listed below twice, flowing into the next exercise without setting the bells down until the end. Be ready!		
Double-Bell Clean p. 56	2	none
Double Front Squat p. 105	2	none
Military Press (2 bells) p. 61 or Seesaw Press p. 62	2	30 sec
Repeat for 3 sets.		

WORKOUT 12 Perform the exercises straight through with little to no rest. Rest 1 minute at the end of each set before performing another set. Once all sets are completed, move on to the next sequence.

Start with Level Three Warm-Up (page 34).		
Exercise	**Reps**	**Rest**
Sequence A		
Tactical Lunge p. 113 or Double-Bell Reverse Lunge p. 111	5 each side	minimal
Double Bent-Over Row p. 92 (You can do pull-ups if you have access to this equipment.)	5–6	minimal
Hand-to-Hand Swing p. 52	20	minimal
Rest/active recovery and repeat 3 rounds.		
Sequence B		
Double-Bell Push-Up p. 77	6	minimal
Sumo Deadlift p. 45	8	minimal
Snatch p. 123 or Double-Bell Snatch p. 124	8	minimal
Rest/active recovery and repeat 3 rounds.		

WORKOUT 13   Perform the Sequence A exercises for the suggested reps. Complete all rounds prior to starting Sequence B.

Exercise	Reps	Rest
Start with Level Three Warm-Up (page 34).		
Sequence A		
1-Arm Swing p. 50	5	minimal
Clean p. 55 and Front Squat p. 105	5	minimal
Double-Bell Push-Up p. 77	5	minimal
High Pull p. 115	5	20–45 sec
Repeat 3 rounds.		
Sequence B Perform 30 seconds of work for each exercise. Break for 30 seconds before moving on to the next. If this isn't challenging enough, shorten the rest to 20 seconds. If it's too challenging, add 15 seconds to the rest portion.		
Snatch (alternating sides) p. 123	30 sec	30 sec
Wide-Leg High Plank p. 87	30 sec	30 sec
2-Arm Swing p. 49	30 sec	30 sec
Deck Squat p. 108	30 sec	30 sec
Janda Sit-Up p. 98	30 sec	30 sec
Pullover to Crunch p. 97	30 sec	30 sec
Repeat 2 rounds.		

WORKOUT 14   Treat the sequences as if they're separate workouts. Rest 1–3 minutes if needed between sequences before moving on to the next.

Start with Level Three Warm-Up (page 34).		
Exercise	**Reps**	**Rest**
Sequence A		
Turkish Get-Up *p. 119*	alternate back and forth for 3 minutes	minimal
Beg: Hot Potato *p. 101* **Int:** Figure 8 *p. 102* **Adv:** Figure 8 to Hold *p. 103*	10 each side 5 each direction 5 each direction	minimal
Sequence B		
Bottoms-Up Clean *p. 59* or Bottoms-Up Press *p. 63*	5 each side	minimal
Single-Leg Deadlift (2 bells) *p. 47*	5 each side	minimal
Double-Bell Dip *p. 79*	5	minimal
Repeat 4 times.		
Sequence C Single-Bell Complex: Staying on one side of the body, perform each exercise once, flowing in to the next exercise. After completing all exercises, repeat on the other side. Perform 3–4 sets on each side if you can.		
1-Arm Swing *p. 50*	1	minimal
Clean *p. 55*	1	minimal
High Pull *p. 115*	1	minimal
Snatch *p. 123*	1	minimal
Set the bell down and rest if needed, otherwise switch to the other side and keep going.		

WORKOUT 15 Perform the Sequence A exercises one after the next with almost no rest. Once you've completed 2–3 rounds, begin Sequence B. Make sure you have your timer ready and are feeling fresh before beginning B.

Start with Level Three Warm-Up (page 34).		
Exercise	**Reps**	**Rest**
Sequence A		
Windmill (Top) p. 72 or Windmill (Double) p. 73	3 each side	minimal
Overhead Squat p. 106	3 each side	minimal
Renegade Row p. 89	3 each side	minimal
Repeat 2 rounds.		
Sequence B Set your timer for 15 seconds of work and 15 seconds of rest. Work very hard to your maximum potential but use your judgment.		
Double Front Squats p. 105	15 sec	15 sec
Double-Bell Push Press p. 64	15 sec	15 sec
Double Swing p. 53	15 sec	15 sec
Double-Bell Clean p. 56	15 sec	15 sec
Alternating Bent-Over Row p. 93	15 sec	15 sec
Snatch (left) p. 123	15 sec	15 sec
Snatch (right) p. 123	15 sec	30–60 sec
Repeat 2–3 rounds, depending on your conditioning level.		

TABATA 3 This is a bonus metabolic conditioning workout. Go through all the exercises for 20 seconds of all-out work and 10 seconds of rest. Start at the top and repeat for a total of 2 sets. As you become more advanced in your fitness, take a 1-minute break after 2 sets and repeat the entire section again for another 2 sets.

Exercise	**Time**	**Sets**	**Rest**
Snatch (left) p. 123	20 sec	2	10 sec
Snatch (right) p. 123	20 sec	2	10 sec
Burpee p. 135	20 sec	2	10 sec
Jumping Jacks p. 136	20 sec	2	10 sec

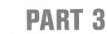

PART 3

The Exercises

Deadlifts

The deadlift is one of the most important exercises to master first. It's the safest way to pick up and put down a kettlebell. If you can't safely perform a deadlift with a kettlebell then you shouldn't move on to any of the ballistic drills such as swings, cleans, and snatches. Learning how to properly pick up a kettlebell off the ground with your hamstrings loaded will carry over into many of your daily activities, such as lifting heavy objects off the floor. This exercise will help strengthen your entire body, starting with your hamstrings, glutes, and abdominals. You'll also be using your lats for the pulling motion. Practice these but never get too comfortable and you'll find yourself getting stronger and stronger.

TIPS FOR ALL DEADLIFTS

• *Don't look down at your feet or the kettlebell because this will allow your lower back to round.*

• *Don't shrug your shoulders up to your ears at the top. Keep your shoulders pulled back and down at the top of the deadlift.*

• *Don't lean back in the standing position.*

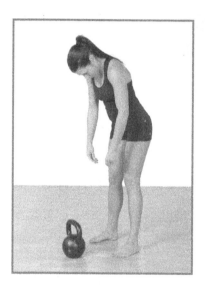 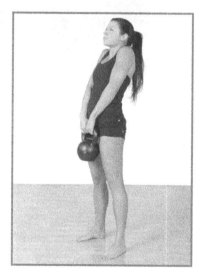 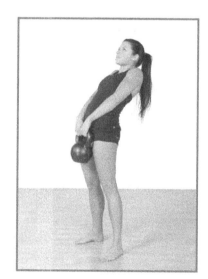

Before diving right into the deadlift or the swing, you need to learn how to hinge from your hips. This movement is extremely important to understand before starting any of the foundation kettlebell exercises.

STARTING POSITION: Stand with your feet shoulder-width apart and find the crease/fold in your hips.

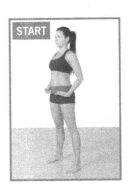

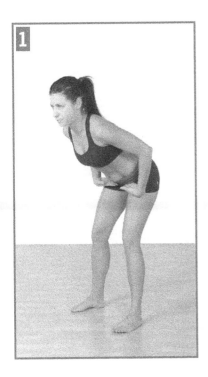

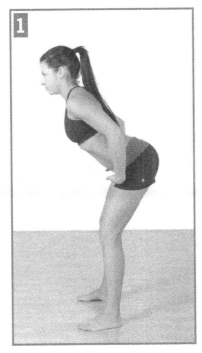

1 Shift your butt back directly behind you as if you were sitting in a high chair. Keep your head straight and maintain a flat back. You should feel a stretch in the backs of your legs and feel as if you can wiggle your toes. *This is not a knee bend or a squat.* Your knees will bend but only because you're reaching your hips back behind you. Stick your butt out! *This is also NOT a back rounding exercise.* (Two views shown.)

This is a prerequisite to learning the swing (page 48).

STARTING POSITION: Stand with your feet shoulder-width apart. Place the kettlebell on the floor between your feet.

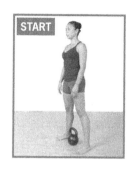

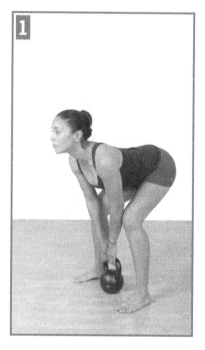

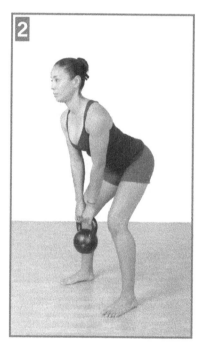

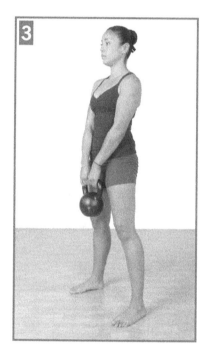

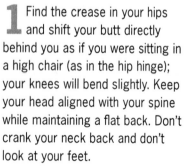 Find the crease in your hips and shift your butt directly behind you as if you were sitting in a high chair (as in the hip hinge); your knees will bend slightly. Keep your head aligned with your spine while maintaining a flat back. Don't crank your neck back and don't look at your feet.

Slowly grab the bell's handle as you actively hinge your hips behind you, keeping your heels planted on the floor.

2–3 Holding the bell in front of you with straight arms, stand up straight, squeezing your glutes at the very top.

DOUBLE-BELL VARIATION:
This can also be done by holding a bell in each hand.

STARTING POSITION: Stand next to the bell with your feet hip-width apart.

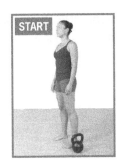
START

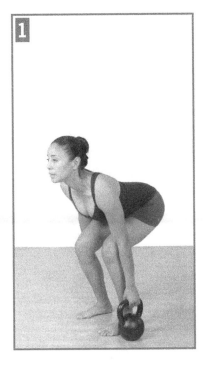

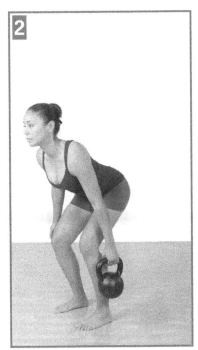

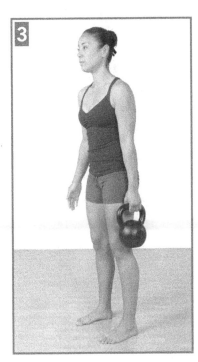

1 Hinge your hips back behind you and grab the handle with one hand. Reach back and down as if you already have two bells in your hands. Use your core so that you don't let the bell pull you to one side.

2–3 Keeping a very flat back and using your legs and glutes, brace your core and pick up the bell. At the top of the movement, keep your shoulders pulled back and down while squeezing your glutes.

STARTING POSITION: Stand between two kettlebells, with your feet no more than hip-width apart.

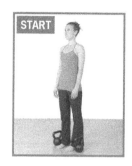

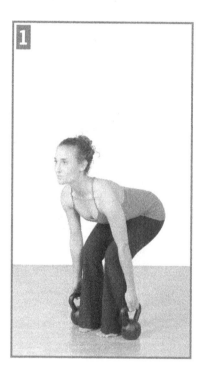

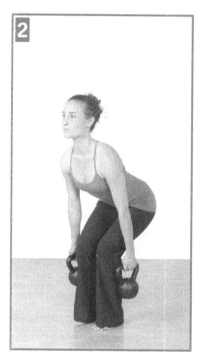

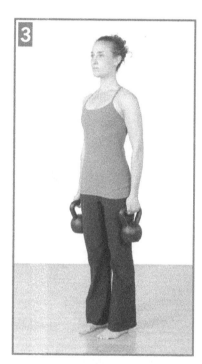

1 Hinge your hips back behind you and grab the handles.

2–3 Using your legs and glutes, brace your core and pick up the bells. At the

top of the movement, keep your shoulders pulled back and down while squeezing your glutes.

This pulling movement can be performed with one or two bells. If you're using very heavy weights, be sure to breathe properly by inhaling through your nose before you lift the bell and exhaling through your teeth or pursed lips on the lift.

STARTING POSITION: Stand with your feet wider than shoulder-width apart, with the bell(s) on the floor between your feet.

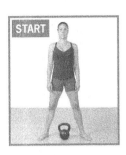

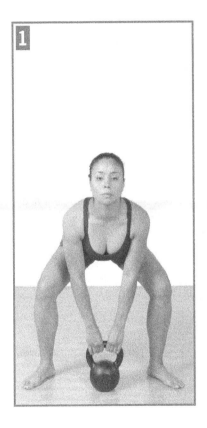

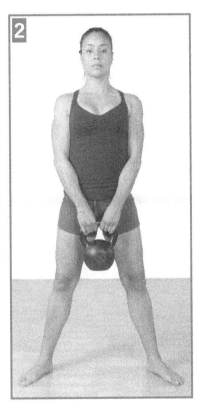

1 Making sure to push you knees slightly open (don't let them bow in), hinge your hips back directly behind you. Keep your head straight while maintaining a flat back. Slowly reach for the bell(s), keeping your knees slightly bent and open as you continue to hinge your hips back behind you.

2 Keeping your heels firmly planted, pick up the bell(s), keeping your arms straight. Stand up straight, squeezing your glutes at the top.

TIP

• Make sure your shoulders don't round forward. Your shoulders should be pulled back and your upper back muscles engaged.

DOUBLE-BELL VARIATION:
This can also be done by holding a bell in each hand.

This is one of my favorite exercises of all time. Upon doing this correctly, your glutes and hamstrings acquire the most amazing strength and thus become very firm. Anytime I feel that things are shifting in the wrong direction, I add this exercise back into my program and immediately my glutes are right where I need them!

Warning: Do not attempt weighted Single-Leg Deadlifts until you've mastered the movement *without* weights. Practice the Single-Leg Deadlift movement BEFORE adding any load. This is a very slow movement—rushing it'll only cause you to fall over.

STARTING POSITION: Ideally you should be barefoot. Stomp one foot in the ground to firmly plant and root it to the floor. Raise your other foot off the ground, keeping your hips parallel and knees facing the same direction. See variations below for kettlebell placement.

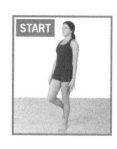

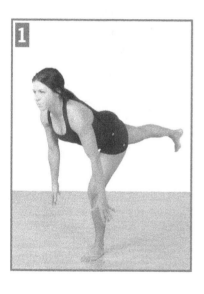

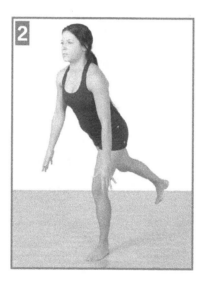

1 Hinge your hips directly back, allowing your raised leg to extend back. Keeping your back flat and engaging your shoulders and lats, inhale and gently reach for the floor or kettlebell. Don't look down at the bell or the floor.

2 Slowly hissing/exhaling, pull yourself up with or without the kettlebell and squeeze the glute of the grounded leg. Your raised leg can continue to be bent or you can gently rest it on the floor if needed.

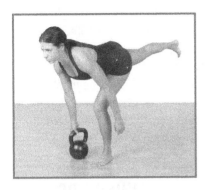

SINGLE-ARM SINGLE-LEG DEADLIFT (CONTRALATERAL): Place the bell outside the foot that will be moving.

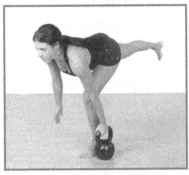

SINGLE-ARM SINGLE-LEG DEADLIFT (BILATERAL): Place the bell on the outside of the grounded foot.

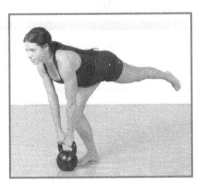

SINGLE BELL IN FRONT: Place the bell right in front of the grounded foot.

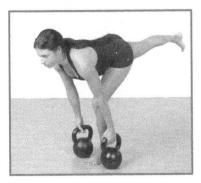

DOUBLE-BELL SINGLE-LEG DEADLIFT: Place two bells on the floor on either side of the grounded foot, with just enough space for the foot to fit between.

Swings

One of the foundation exercises that teaches the powerful hip snap, the swing also conditions and strengthens the entire body. This exercise is at the core of many kettlebell drills and thus carries over to an unlimited number of activities. People have documented losing hundreds of pounds and transforming their entire body with this exercise alone. I personally enjoy variety and balance and that's why I suggest using a multi-faceted amount of proper movements. You can, however, get close to a full-body workout using just the swing. Take the most time mastering this drill and you'll be very pleased with your overall results. If you ever get overwhelmed with too many exercises, you can always go back to doing swings. Even after performing kettlebell swings for seven years, I continue to find ways to make them better and more efficient. The key is to never get too comfortable!

TIPS FOR ALL SWING VARIATIONS

• *Don't hike the kettlebell back too low to the ground. Your forearms need to be close to the groin to avoid using your back.*

• *Don't look down at your feet. This will cause your back to round, which can easily lead to injury.*

• *Don't let the bell droop down at the top of the swing. The bell should be an extension of your arm and needs to be parallel to the ground at the top of the swing. If the bell is drooping then your hips may not be doing the work and your shoulders are probably taking over.*

• *Don't lean back at the very top of the swing. This puts too much pressure on your lower back and won't allow abdominal contraction.*

• *Don't collapse like an accordion and bend your knees first. It's a hip hinge, not a squat!*

• *Don't allow your shoulders to become your new earrings! Keep your shoulders pulled back and down so that you don't injure them or your neck. By using your neck and shoulders during the swing, you'll completely take away the purpose of using your hips. Remember: This is a hip, glute, and core exercise—not a shoulder exercise!*

BREATHING TIPS

When performing ballistic exercises such as swings, cleans, and snatches, sharply inhale or sniff through your nose as you actively hike the bell and your hips back. Use a fast power breath "hiss" as you snap and thrust your hips forward. When the bell reaches the top of the swing, you should feel your core bracing due to the powerful breath you released during each hip thrust. Your breath should be in sync with the movement.

STARTING POSITION: Stand with your feet between hip- and shoulder-width apart and the bell on the floor about 12 inches in front of you. Hinge your hips back, keeping a slight bend in your knees. Keeping your back flat, grab the bell's handle with both hands and tilt it slightly toward you. This movement loads your hamstrings and engages your lats for optimal swing performance.

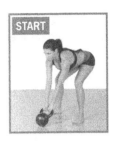

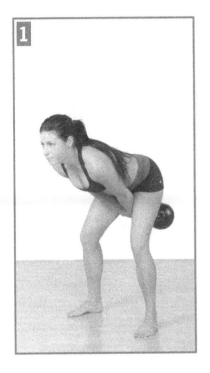

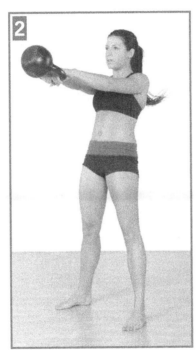

1 Hike the bell through your legs with power while keeping it close to your upper inner thighs.

2 Thrust your hips forward, quickly clench your glutes, and lock out your legs to a standing position. The bell should float up due to the power that your hips create. Make sure during the thrust that you're driving through your heels while keeping them planted on the floor. At the top of the swing, shrink your abdominals by bringing your rib cage closer to your belly button. *Note:* Don't hyperextend your knees, but gently lock them for optimal power.

Continue hiking the bell and your hips back at the same time and then thrusting your hips forward to the standing position for multiple reps.

Don't let your body twist when using only one arm. It should look just as smooth and crisp as the 2-Arm Swing (page 49).

STARTING POSITION: Stand with your feet between hip- and shoulder-width apart and the bell on the floor about 12 inches in front of you. Hinge your hips back behind you, keeping a slight bend in your knees. Keeping your back flat, grab the bell's handle with one hand. Make sure your shoulder stays in its socket and tilt the bell slightly toward you, activating your lats.

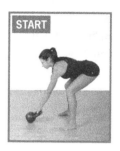

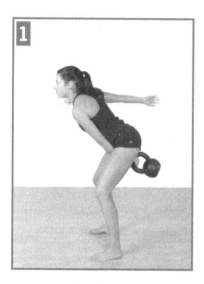

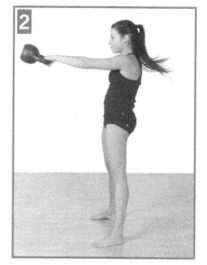

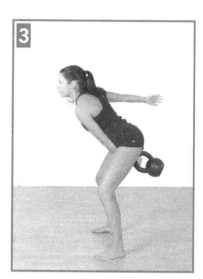

1 Hike the bell back through your legs while actively hinging back. The bell should be swung close to the tops of your inner thighs while your free hand swings along the outside of your body.

2 Driving through your heels, thrust your hips forward to a standing position while keeping your feet firmly planted on the floor; bring your knee caps up by locking them out. Your quads should be very tight! The bell should float up from the power that your hips create. Squeeze your glutes once you reach the standing position. Your free arm should mimic your working arm throughout the swing. At the top, have your free hand tap the bell.

Note: Shrink your abdominals at the top of the swing by bringing your rib cage toward your belly button.

3 Actively hike the bell and your hips back at the same time with power, keeping your forearm very close to your groin.

Continue thrusting your hips forward to the standing position and hiking your hips back for multiple reps.

TIP

- When performing the 1-Arm Swing, stay in control by keeping your shoulder pulled back and down. Don't chase the bell by letting it pull your shoulder out of its socket, thus bringing your torso out of alignment.

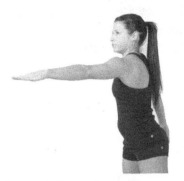

Incorrect alignment

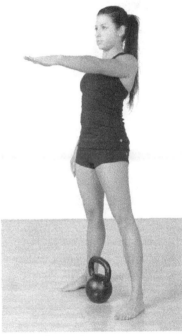

Proper alignment

This exercise not only has all the benefits of the swing, but it adds the hand-eye coordination component that may allow you to forget how hard you're actually working.

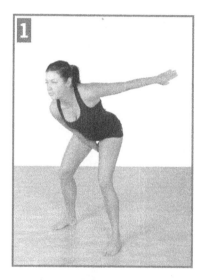

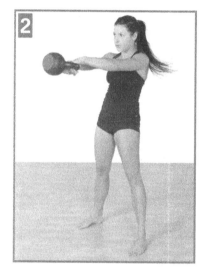

1 Start the 1-Arm Swing. Have your free hand mirror your working hand to get it ready for the pass.

2 At the top of the swing, around chest level, pass the bell off to your free hand. Don't forget to keep your hip thrusts and breath powerful as you change hands.

HAND-TO-HAND (H2H) SWING VARIATION: It's important to be very comfortable with the Alternating Swing before attempting this more-advanced version. Be sure to practice on grass or soft sand just in case you drop the bell. During the pass, take your hand off the bell at the very top of the swing and have your free hand ready to catch the bell in mid-air. The bell will be airborne for a split second and your free hand will catch the bell on the switch.

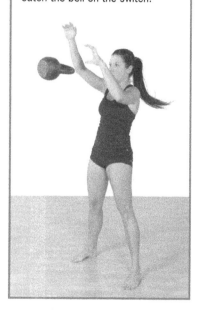

Be sure your form is perfect with all of the previous swings before attempting this one.

STARTING POSITION: Place two even-sized kettlebells on the floor in front of you with the handles slightly pointing back. The handles will create a "V" shape. You may want to take a slightly wider stance than with the single bell since you'll be passing two bells between your legs. Hinge your hips back, keeping a slight bend in your knees, and grab the handles. Remember to keep your back flat.

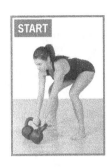

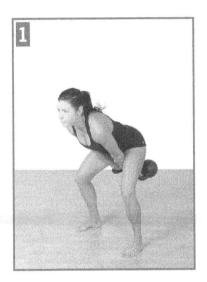

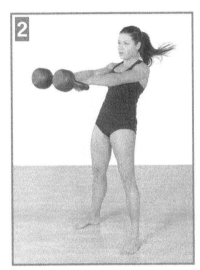

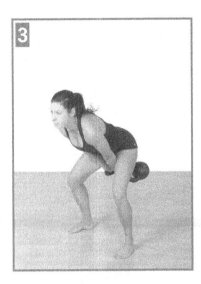

1 Hike the bells back behind you with your thumbs pointing back slightly.

2 Thrust your hips forward and straighten out the bells at the very top. Don't try to raise the bells and lean back. Stand tall at the top of the swing and let your legs and hips power the bells up. If the bells end up between belly button and chest height, you performed a solid rep.

3 Hike the bells and your hips back again to repeat. Make sure the weight of the bells is being absorbed by your hamstrings and not your back.

Cleans

Used in many other kettlebell drills as well as being an exercise in itself, the clean is primarily used to teach you how to safely bring the kettlebell up to rack position. There are several different styles of cleans; this book teaches you the most current way that the Russian Kettlebell Challenge (RKC), the first and original kettlebell certification system, practices. If you have sensitive wrists or forearms, you may want to consider wrist bands or wrist protection until you perfect the form.

The rack position is where the kettlebell ends up when you clean the bell. The kettlebell should rest on the outside of the forearm, gently brushed up against the shoulder. The wrist should be in neutral position with the palm all the way through the handle of the bell. The hand should have a very relaxed grip on the handle. The shoulder should be down and the elbow close to the body. Get very comfortable with the rack position. A weak rack position will hinder you from being able to do other kettlebell lifts smoothly.

Note that you can also grip the handle of the bell from a diagonal angle so that the handle is resting deep inside the palm of your hand. This will avoid the bending back of the wrist.

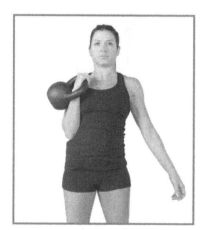 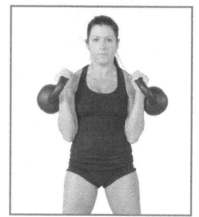

Examples of proper rack position

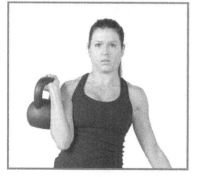 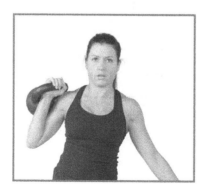 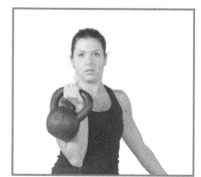

Examples of bad rack positions from left to right: Hand and kettlebell are too far outside the body; elbow should be hugging the body, not flared out; kettlebell is too far forward, elbow is too close inside.

Your legs and hips are the driving force behind cleaning the bell.

STARTING POSITION: Stand with your feet hip-width apart and the bell in front of you with the handle positioned diagonally. Hinge your hips back and grab the handle the same way you would when starting the 1-Arm Swing (page 50). Your thumb should be pointed toward your body.

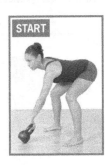

START

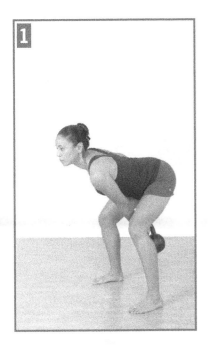

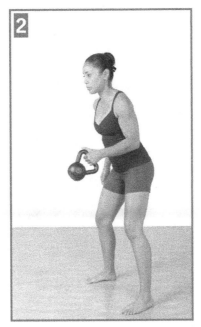

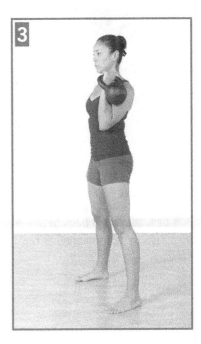

1 Actively hinging back your hips, hike the bell behind you with your thumb leading.

2–3 Thrust your hips forward while rotating the bell around your forearm and up to rack position, loosening your grip as you rotate the bell in your hand. Your hand should be far inside the

handle. Make sure to rack the bell on the outside of your breast. The bell should be held tightly against the shoulder and your wrist should be straight.

continued on next page

continued from previous page

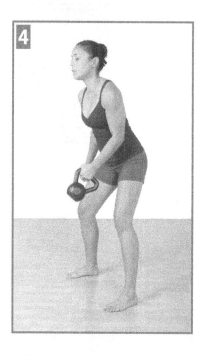

4 Loosen your grip, unwind the bell, and hike it back between your legs to perform another rep.

TIPS

• Don't swing your arm far away from your body as if doing the 1-Arm Swing. Keep your elbow as close to your body as possible during the active portion of the movement. This is called "taming the arc."

• Don't bend your wrist back in rack position. The wrist needs to be straight for all rack positions.

• Don't use your biceps during the clean—this is not a biceps curl! The power should come from your hips.

MODIFICATION: If you have problems "taming the arc," try performing the clean facing a wall. This will quickly teach you to keep your arm closer to your body, rather than let it run wild away from you.

DOUBLE-BELL VARIATION: The clean can also be done with two bells. Have the kettlebells in front of you on the floor with the handles forming a "V" shape.

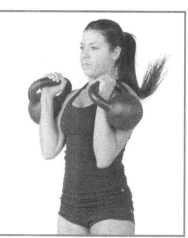

This method is primarily used in kneeling or seated exercises to get the bell safely to rack position. Beginners can use this method if they're having a difficult time mastering the clean from the standing position.

STARTING POSITION: Sit on the floor with straight legs, kneel, or stand. The kettlebell is directly in front of you on the floor. If you're sitting, your legs should straddle the bell.

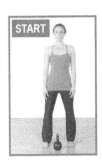
START

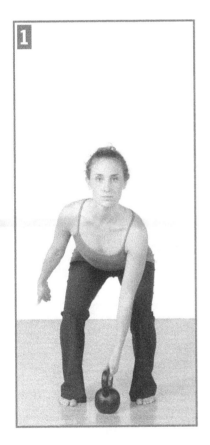

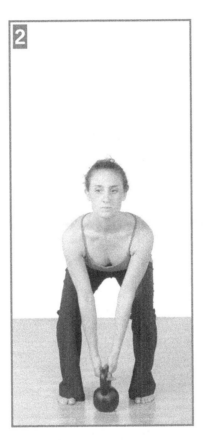

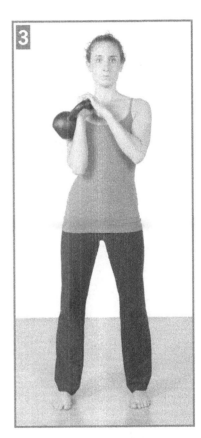

1 Place your left hand through the handle.

2 Place your right hand through the handle over your left hand.

3 Using both arms, bring the kettlebell to rack position on the right side.

Switch hand placements to cheat curl the bell to rack position on the other side.

STARTING POSITION: Stand with your feet hip-width apart and the bell in rack position.

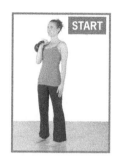

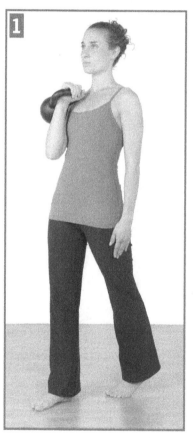

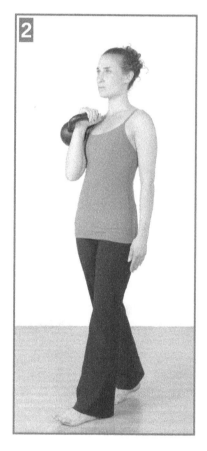

DOUBLE-BELL VARIATION: This excellent core exercise can also be done with two bells. Make sure to keep both shoulders down. Work your way up to a minute.

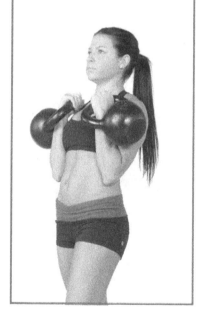

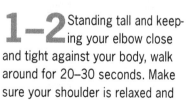 Standing tall and keeping your elbow close and tight against your body, walk around for 20–30 seconds. Make sure your shoulder is relaxed and your posture is upright. Your wrist should always remain in neutral position.

Repeat on both sides.

Use a lighter kettlebell when you first start learning this exercise.

STARTING POSITION: Stand with your feet roughly hip-width apart with a kettlebell and its handle set vertically between your feet. Hinge your hips back, loading your hamstrings to prepare for hiking the bell, and reach for the handle with your thumb facing forward, away from your body.

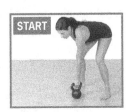

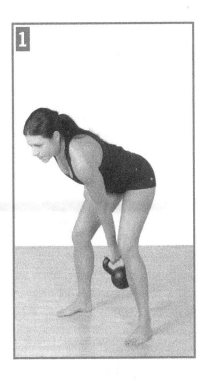

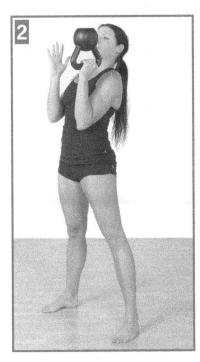

1 Hike the bell behind you.

2 Crush the handle of the bell by squeezing it very hard as you thrust your hips to a locked-out position. Keeping your elbow close to your body, bring the ball of the bell right side up to rack position. Make sure to tense your lats, biceps, core, and glutes at the top of this clean. Keep your free hand close by to protect your face in case you don't have proper control of the bell.

Loosen your hand and hike the bell back for another rep.

Overhead Presses

Most people think of the press as just a shoulder exercise; however, this is not just a shoulder exercise. When you use the correct breathing and tension while tightening all of the muscles throughout your body, you'll find your muscles working as a team to get the kettlebell safely over your head. Heavier weights will be easier to press overhead, without injury, if you utilize proper tension throughout your body.

Warning: If you have any shoulder or thoracic mobility restrictions or pain, be sure to get that taken care of before attempting any overhead lifts. Spend extra time with the thoracic and shoulder mobility drills. You'll only make your condition worse if your form is compromised.

When the bell is pressed overhead, like in the Military Press, you should be in *overhead lockout position:* elbow locked, triceps engaged, wrist straight, palm facing forward, shoulder pulled down into the socket, and lat muscle flared out for extra stability. The bell should be slightly behind your head and your biceps aligned with your ear.

MILITARY PRESS

STARTING POSITION: Stand with your feet hip-width apart and the bell in rack position.

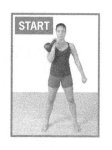

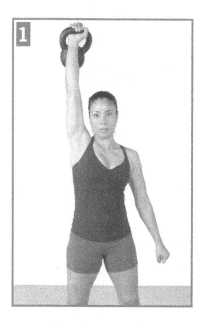

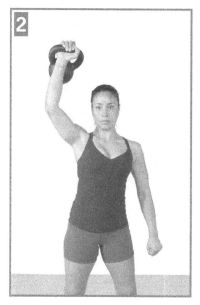

1 Squeezing your glutes and locking out your legs, press the bell up to overhead lockout position. Make sure to press the bell up in one straight line rather than bringing your elbow way out to the side.

2 Pull the bell down using your lat muscle, slowly lowering your elbow back to the rack position rather than letting gravity take over.

From here, you can clean the bell again before performing another rep for a slight break or just squeeze your glutes and press the bell back up to overhead lockout position.

TIPS

• Don't bend your wrist.

• Don't lean back or tilt your head back at the top of the press in order to force the kettlebell to be vertical. This will put pressure on your back and won't help your tight shoulders or thoracic mobility restrictions.

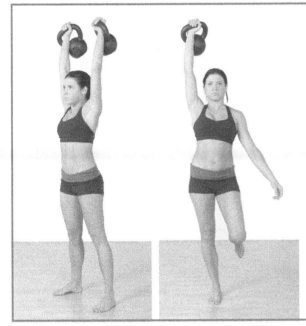

DOUBLE-BELL VARIATION: This can also be done with two bells. Make sure that your palms face forward in the top position while your shoulders remain retracted and packed down.

SINGLE-LEG VARIATION: This advanced move has the bell on the same side as the stabilizing leg.

Squeeze your glute and engage your quad by bringing your knee cap up. You'll also squeeze the handle and use the power breath while pushing the bell up overhead.

STARTING POSITION: Stand with your feet hip-width apart and a bell in each hand in rack position.

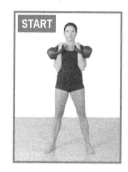

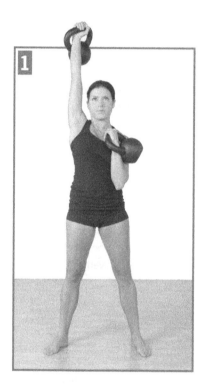

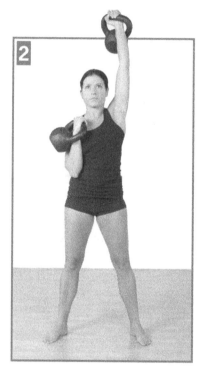

1 Squeeze your glutes and press one of the kettlebells up to overhead lockout position. Tense your glutes for the majority of the time in order to protect your lower back.

2 Similar to a seesaw movement, pull the kettlebell back down to rack position while pressing the other bell up.

Only attempt this after you've mastered the Bottoms-Up Clean (page 59). Use a lighter kettlebell when you first start learning this exercise.

STARTING POSITION: Stand with your feet roughly hip-width apart with a kettlebell set vertically between your feet. Hinge your hips and place one hand on the handle.

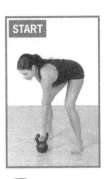

START

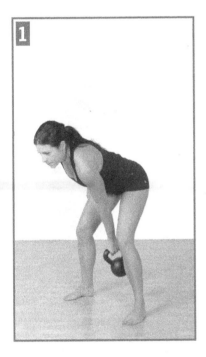

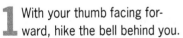

1 With your thumb facing forward, hike the bell behind you.

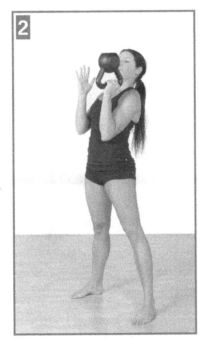

2 Crush the handle of the bell by squeezing it very hard as you thrust your hips forward to the Bottoms-Up Clean lockout position. Your lat is completely engaged and your entire body is tense. Keep your free hand close by in order to protect your face in case you lose control of the bell.

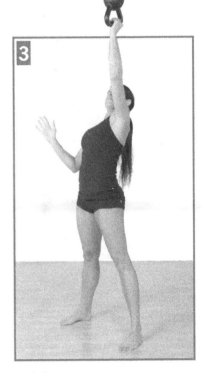

3 Keeping your eyes on the bell and your free hand close by the whole time, press the bell upward using your lats.

Lower it down with control back to the Bottoms-Up Clean position, or hike it back for another Bottoms-Up Clean before pressing it back up.

The push press is a great exercise that uses the power in your legs to press the kettlebell over your head. It can also quickly become a conditioning exercise if done with high reps and/or for speed.

STARTING POSITION: Stand with your feet hip-width apart and the bell in rack position.

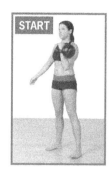

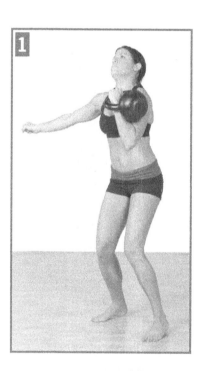

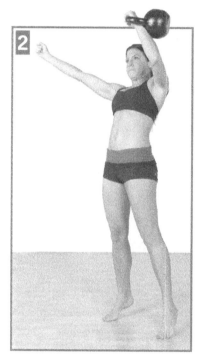

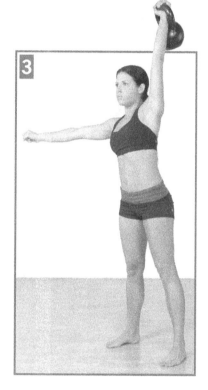

1 Dip by bending your knees slightly and lowering your hips.

2–3 Drive your hips up explosively while punching the bell up to lockout position.

Lower the bell down and immediately dip again for continuous, explosive reps.

DOUBLE-BELL VARIATION: This can also be done with two bells.

Only perform this exercise if you can sit on the floor without slouching and rounding your lower back.

STARTING POSITION: Sit on the floor with your legs straight and straddling the bell on the floor.

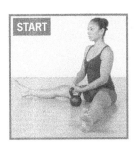

START

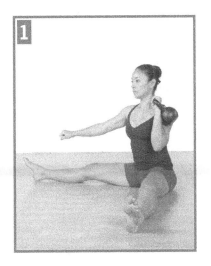

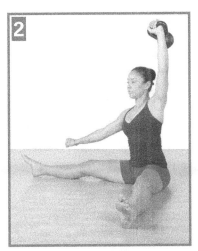

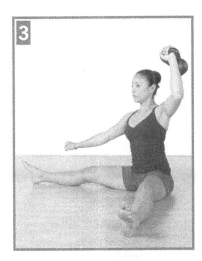

1 Cheat curl (see page 57) the bell to rack position.

2 Crush the bell by firmly squeezing the handle and press it to overhead lockout position. Make a fist with your free hand to create more tension for the working side.

3 Slowly return the bell to rack position.

STARTING POSITION: Kneel tall on a soft pad with your shoulders and hips stacked in alignment. The kettlebell should be on the floor in front of your knees.

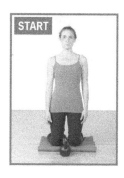

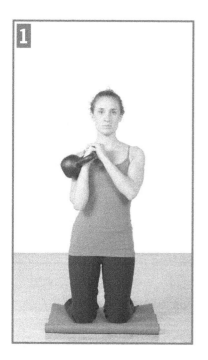

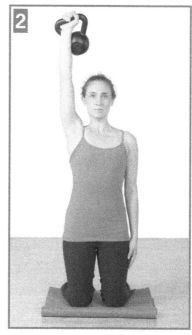

1 Cheat curl (see page 57) the bell to the rack position.

2 Tense your glutes and press the kettlebell to overhead lockout position.

STARTING POSITION: Kneel on a soft pad with one leg stepped out in front of you as if for a lunge.

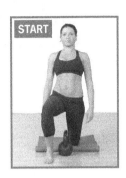

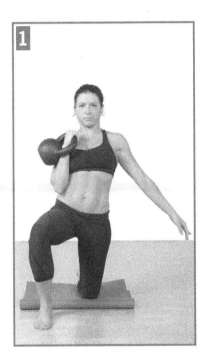

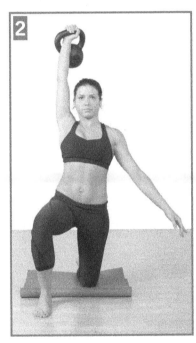

1 Cheat curl (see page 57) the bell to the rack position on the side where the foot is stepped forward.

2 Tense your glutes and press the kettlebell to overhead lockout position.

This is an excellent exercise for posture and shoulder stability.

STARTING POSITION: Stand with the kettlebell in overhead lockout position with your palm facing forward.

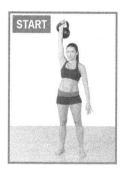

START

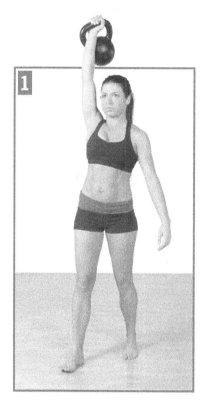

1 Making sure your lats are flared out to help with the stabilization of the bell, walk around with the bell overhead. Work up to 30 seconds.

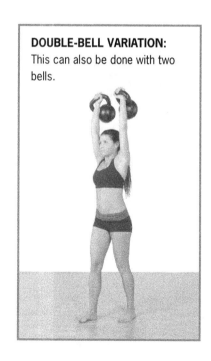

DOUBLE-BELL VARIATION: This can also be done with two bells.

Windmills

An excellent drill for shoulders, hips, and obliques, the windmill will teach you mobility, strength, focus, and body awareness. This is an advanced exercise so be sure to use a lighter weight when first attempting the lower or upper windmills. When you do start adding weights to your windmills, be sure to keep the reps low.

TIPS FOR ALL WINDMILLS

- *Don't round your back just to touch the floor. If you're not flexible, don't force yourself to touch the floor—go through the motion as far as your hips allow.*

- *Don't rush through this exercise.*

- *Don't shift forward on your front leg as you reach for the floor. Treat your front leg as a kickstand—most of your weight needs to be focused on your back leg.*

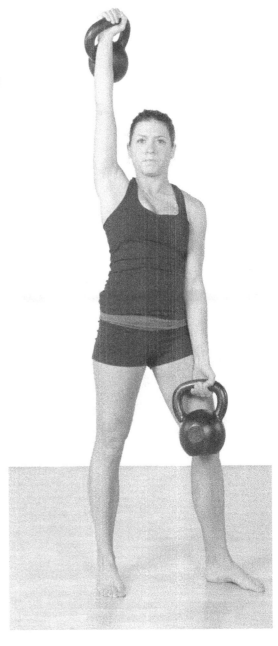

STARTING POSITION: Stand with your feet hip-width apart and pointing to your right at roughly a 45-degree angle. Raise your left hand up to the ceiling.

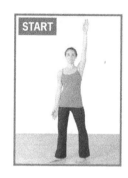

START

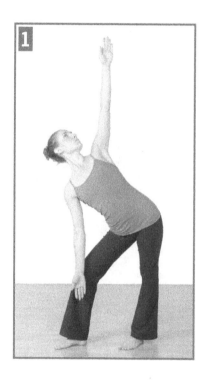

1

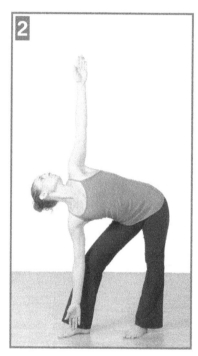

2

1 Keeping your left leg locked and your eye on your upper hand throughout the exercise, hinge your hips out to the left.

2 With a slight bend in your right leg, reach your right hand toward the floor. Be sure to keep most of the weight on your back leg; the front leg is just your kickstand.

This is the easiest weighted version.

STARTING POSITION: Stand with your feet hip-width apart and pointing to your right at roughly a 45-degree angle. Place a bell on the floor just inside the instep of your right foot. Raise your left hand and keep an eye on it throughout the exercise. Hinge your hips out to the left.

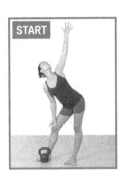

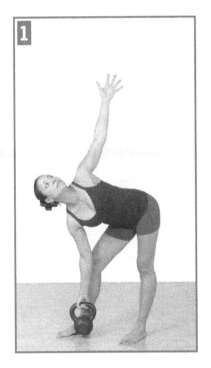

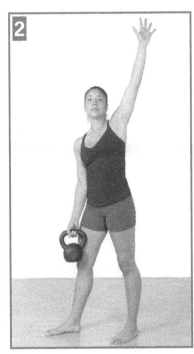

1 Inhale to brace your core as you reach down for the kettlebell. You can allow your shoulder to rotate a bit as you make your descent.

2 Exhale slowly and squeeze your left glute on your way up to the standing position.

This is the intermediate version. Remember: Your shoulder can rotate around as you move your body throughout the windmill—you're moving around the bell.

STARTING POSITION: Stand with your feet hip-width apart and pointing to your right at roughly a 45-degree angle. With your left hand, bring the kettlebell to overhead lockout position; your arm should be perpendicular to the floor throughout the movement.

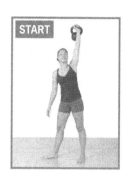

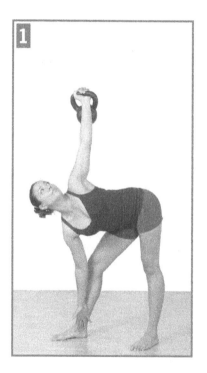

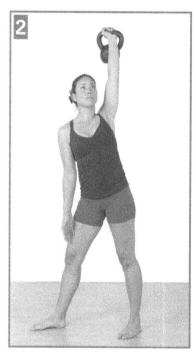

1 Keeping your eyes on the bell at all times, hinge your hips out to the left, inhale, and slowly reach for the floor.

2 Keeping the bell and shoulder packed, exhale slowly and stand back up.

Before you complete another rep, make sure that your shoulder remains pulled down and packed.

WINDMILL (DOUBLE)

This is the most advanced version because it combines the bottom and top windmills. Only attempt this after mastering the other windmills, which can take several weeks to months. Be patient! Note that you don't need to have two even-sized bells for this exercise. When just beginning, the top bell can be much lighter than the bottom bell. Staying tight with your breathing will be very important, especially when you start loading more weight.

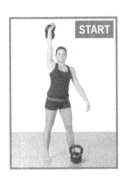

STARTING POSITION: Stand with your feet hip-width apart and pointing to your left at roughly a 45-degree angle. Place one kettlebell on the floor just inside your left foot. With your right hand, bring another kettlebell to overhead lockout position; your arm should be perpendicular to the floor throughout the movement.

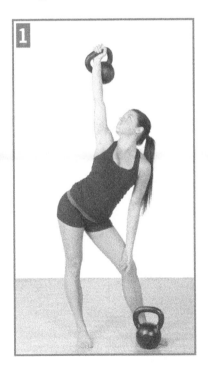

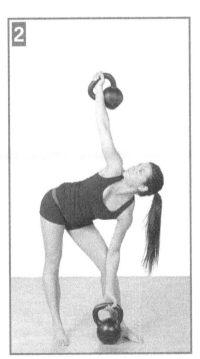

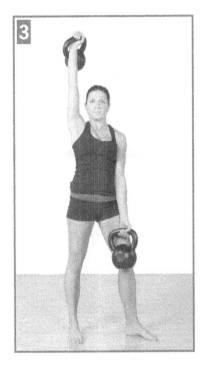

1–2 Keeping your eye on the overhead bell at all times, windmill your body down and reach for the bottom bell with your palm facing away from you.

3 Pick up the bottom bell by windmilling your body back up to the standing position.

For another rep, hinge your hips to the right and slowly bring the bottom kettlebell back to the inside of your left foot.

Push-Ups

Push-ups are an amazing exercise when done correctly. Unfortunately, most women don't practice push-ups diligently and therefore lack the upper body strength and core connection. Most people learn to do wider push-ups, which place more emphasis on the chest and shoulders. This is probably a big reason why women shy away from this exercise. In my opinion, wider push-ups should only be done from time to time because doing too many is a sure-fire way to trash your shoulders. By keeping your hands closer together and your elbows close to your sides, you're using more triceps and are thus able to engage your lats more easily. This is a much safer and more effective way to practice push-ups. Push-ups are a very effective abdominal exercise as well because you have to stabilize and brace your core in order to protect your back. If you feel your lower back start to sway, stop immediately or practice on a higher surface (such as a stable bench or counter).

Before performing push-ups on kettlebells, make sure that you're capable of properly executing them with your hands on the ground. Always check that you're using two very stable kettlebells. Bells smaller than 12kg (25lb) should not be used due to their instability. The heavier the bell, the more stable it is. Not only does this style of push-up work your core, triceps, shoulders, and back, it'll strengthen your hands and wrists.

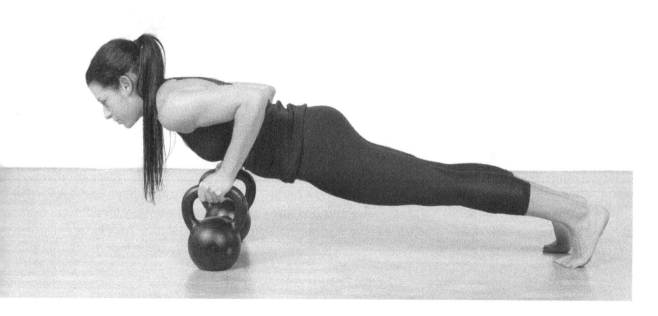

BODYWEIGHT PUSH-UP

Before you start doing push-ups on kettlebells, make sure you can perform them properly on just your hands. Soon you'll be ready for some awesome full-range push-ups on kettlebells to further your push-up progression. *Important:* Don't let your lower body fall toward the ground. Keep it tight!

Breathing for push-ups: Inhale as you lower yourself down and then exhale quickly and powerfully to brace your core as you push yourself up.

STARTING POSITION: Assume a high plank, with hands on the floor, wrists completely underneath your shoulders, and toes on the ground. Your body should form a diagonal line from head to feet.

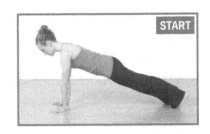

START

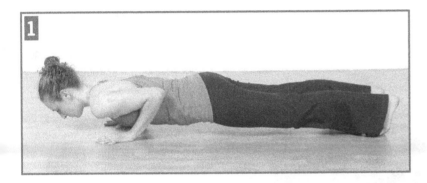

1

1 Inhaling, bend your elbows back and keep them along your sides to lower your entire body toward the floor. If you're advanced, your nose should be able to touch the floor; otherwise, just lower halfway. Keep your entire core and back tight throughout the down and up motion.

2 Exhaling, push through your palms and engage your triceps to raise yourself back up.

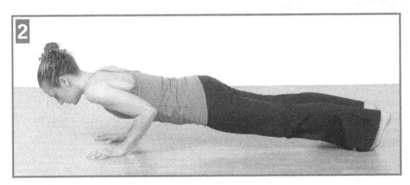

2

MODIFICATION: This can also be done on your knees until you get stronger, or you can place your hands on a higher surface (such as a stable table or chair seat).

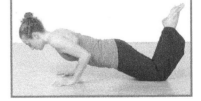

Push-Ups | **75**

Even if you can do push-ups from your toes, you should practice kettlebell push-ups from your knees first to get used to the balance involved. You may use a mat for your knees.

STARTING POSITION: Place the upright kettlebells shoulder-width apart, directly underneath your shoulders, and prop yourself up on them. Your hands should be wrapped around each handle directly on the center for extra stability; keep your wrists in neutral position. Make sure that your arms are locked. Step your knees behind you so that your body forms a straight line from head to knees.

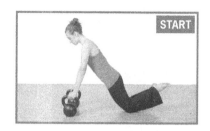

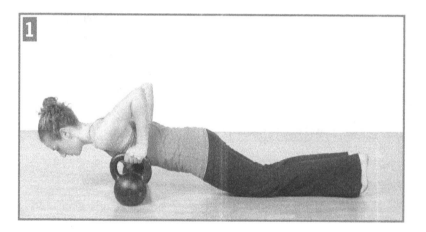

1 Take a breath in to brace your core and slowly lower your body down toward the floor. Bend your elbows back, keeping them along your sides.

2 Push your body up using your triceps, shoulders, and core muscles. Remember to exhale on the way up.

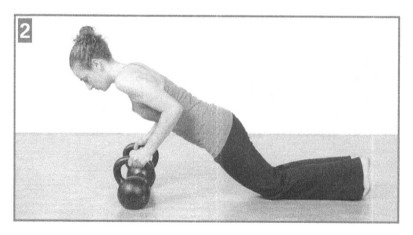

MODIFICATION: If you don't have a pair of larger kettlebells, place each hand on a yoga block or bench.

DOUBLE-BELL PUSH-UP

STARTING POSITION: Place the upright kettlebells shoulder-width apart, directly underneath your shoulders, and prop yourself up on them. Your hands should be wrapped around each handle directly on the center for extra stability; keep your wrists in neutral position. Make sure that your arms are locked. Step your feet behind you so that your body forms a straight line from head to heel. This is the high plank position on kettlebells.

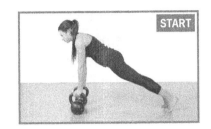

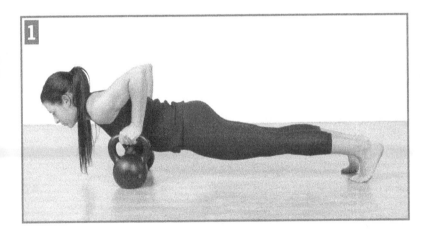

1 Inhaling, slowly bend your elbows back and keep your arms along your sides to lower your entire body to the floor. If you're really strong, you should almost be able to touch your chest to the ground. If not, just lower yourself halfway down.

2 Exhaling, push through your triceps, lats, and shoulders to raise yourself back up to the high plank position.

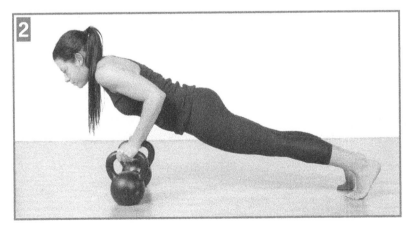

Bells heavier than 8kg work best.

STARTING POSITION: Place a kettlebell on its side with the handle touching the ground, pointed away from you. Assume a high plank position with legs shoulder-width apart and both hands wrapped around the handle of the bell.

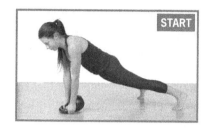

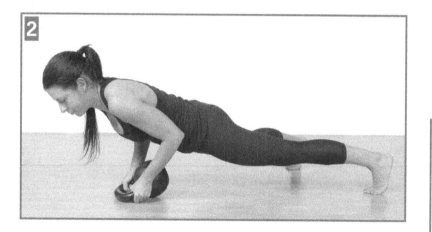

1 Slowly lower your body while letting your elbows flare out slightly.

2 Push yourself back up to the starting position.

MODIFICATION: If you have a hard time stabilizing yourself on the bell, place your knees on the floor.

DOUBLE-BELL DIP

STARTING POSITION: Place yourself between two push-up-sized kettle-bells that you can comfortably stabilize on with your legs extended out in front of you. Grip a handle in each hand.

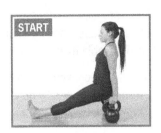

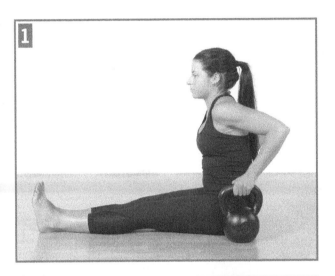

1 While keeping your spine erect, lower your body by bending your elbows back behind you until they're parallel to the floor.

2 Using your triceps and shoulders, straighten your arms while lifting your bottom off the floor.

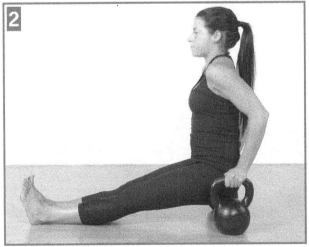

MODIFICATION: To make this easier, bend your legs so that they can assist with the dipping motion.

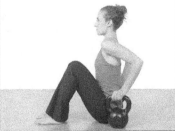

Floor Presses

Floor presses are done slowly with control while lying flat on your back. This great strength exercise targets your chest, triceps, shoulders, and core muscles, which all work together to press the bell up. With proper tension, you'll be able to engage almost all of your muscles, including your lats and quadriceps.

In this section, you'll learn how to properly bring the kettlebell(s) in toward your body for a safe start. The floor presses are generally done with the legs straight and roughly shoulder-width apart, but if you suffer from chronic lower back issues, you may want to bend your knees and place your feet flat on the floor.

TIPS

• *Think about driving yourself into the ground rather than pushing the bell up with your shoulder. You'll be able to move heavier bells once you learn to get your entire body working in concert.*

• *Brace your core with a power breath.*

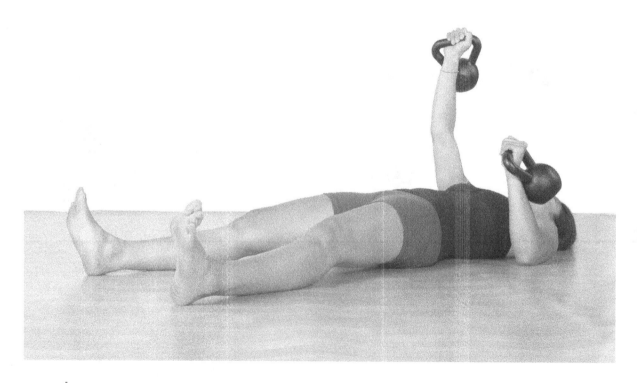

STARTING POSITION: Lie flat on the floor with a kettlebell on the floor next to one side of your torso.

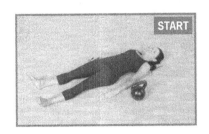

START

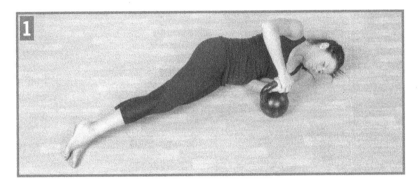

1

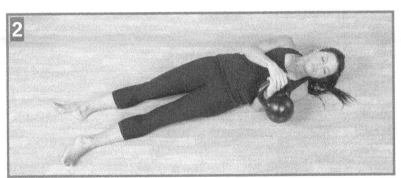

2

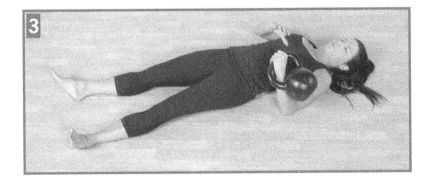

3

1 Roll your entire body toward the kettlebell and place your bottom hand through the handle and your top hand over the handle.

2–3 Keeping the bell close to your torso, roll your body back to starting position. The kettlebell will be gently resting on your forearm in a modified rack position with your wrist straight.

Be sure to roll back over to your side to set the bell down.

STARTING POSITION: Lie flat on the floor with a kettlebell on the floor on either side of your torso.

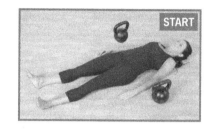

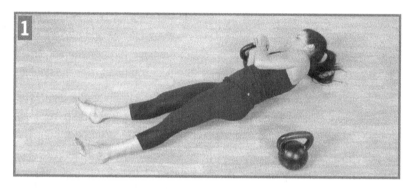

1 Roll your entire body toward your slightly weaker arm.

2–3 Use the pick-up method for 1 bell on this side, then roll gently toward the other side while keeping the bell in rack position.

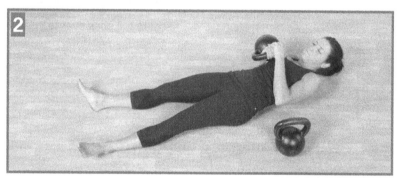

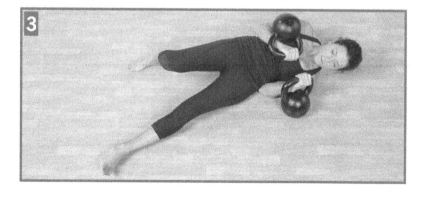

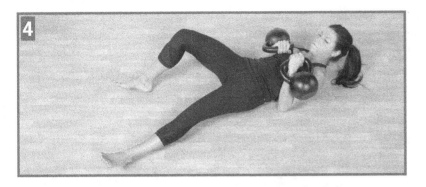

4–5 Keeping both bells in rack position, curl or roll the other bell in very tight toward your body so that you're now ready to perform double kettlebell floor exercises.

Be sure to roll back over to either side to set the bells down.

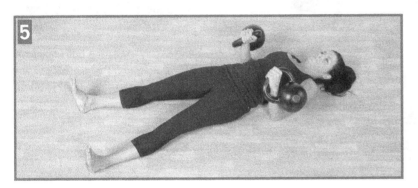

STARTING POSITION: Lie flat on your back with your thighs engaged and your toes pointed at the ceiling. Hold the kettlebell by the ball of the bell with the handle between the index finger and thumb of both hands. Position the bell a few inches above your chest.

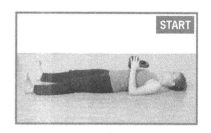

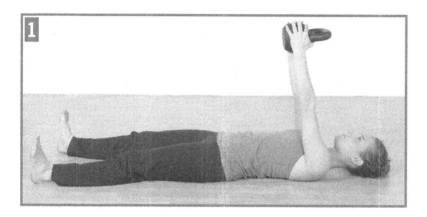

1 Press the bell up until your arms are fully locked but not hyperextended.

2 Slowly lower the bell until your arms touch the ground and are very close to your sides.

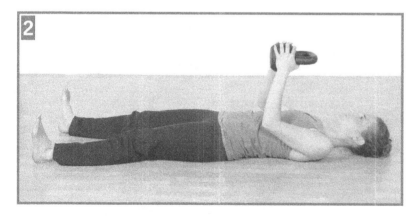

STARTING POSITION: Lie flat on your back with your legs shoulder-width apart. Use the Floor Side Roll Pick-Up Method (1 Bell) (page 81) to get one bell into position. Your free hand should be comfortably off to the side, about a 45-degree angle away from your body.

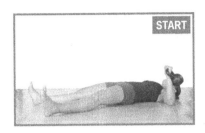

START

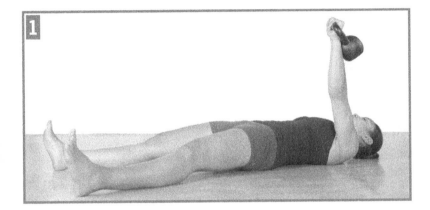

1 Keeping the bell on the outside of your wrist, press it up until your arm is fully extended and locked out over your chest. Power breathe as you press up to activate your core and prevent the bell from pulling you over to one side. Make a fist with your free hand for added tension. This extra tension will help you progress to heavier kettlebells.

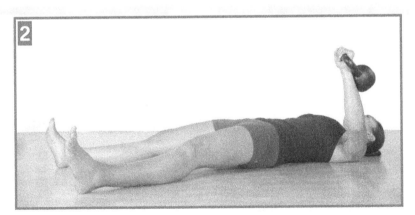

2 Maintaining the vertical alignment of the bell, slowly lower your elbow back down toward the floor.

DOUBLE-BELL VARIATION:
This can also be done with two bells. Use the Floor Side Roll Pick-Up Method (2 Bells) (page 82) to get two bells into position, then think about pushing yourself into the ground as you press both bells up. For constant core pressure, remember to power breathe during each rep. Keep your elbows close to your sides at the bottom, no farther out than 45-degree angles.

STARTING POSITION: Lie flat on your back with your legs shoulder width-apart. Use the Floor Side Roll Pick-Up Method (2 Bells) (page 82) to get two bells into position.

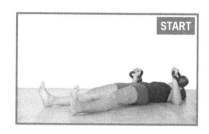

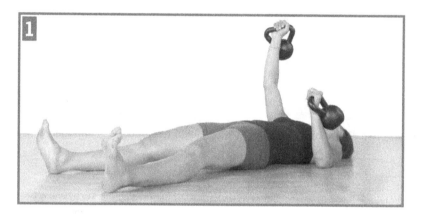

1 Press one kettlebell up to the lockout position over your chest.

2 As you pull the first bell down, press the other up. Think of your arms like a seesaw.

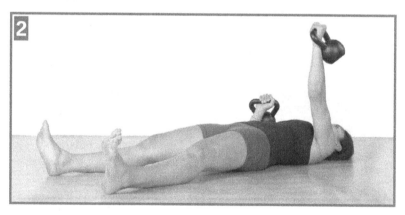

Rows

It's easy to forget about pulling exercises. Many people just like to work the muscles they can visually see and therefore forget about the posterior chain. Most new clients that come to see me lack the proper back muscles. Their shoulders are rounded forward and their chest is practically fused together from being so tight. Meanwhile, their back muscles are stretched out and taut, often causing pain that can radiate up to the neck. Desk jobs, sitting too much, and long bouts at the computer will do that to you very quickly!

The next group of exercises is dedicated to getting the pull that everyone needs. I highly suggest you get a hold of some type of apparatus (like a suspension trainer or pull-up bar) so that you can start learning to pull your own body weight. For the sake of this book, we'll stick to kettlebell exercises that incorporate rowing and pulling. For a complete and well-balanced body, however, you should integrate pulling your own body weight horizontally and vertically into your exercise routine.

RENEGADE ROW PREP

The Renegade Row is a fabulous core, shoulder, triceps, and full-back exercise that'll give you a lot of bang for your buck. Take your time with the following three pre-exercises that will prepare you for the full Renegade Row (page 89). Make sure you can correctly complete each of these before attempting the Renegade Row.

STEP 1: WIDE-LEG HIGH PLANK

This high plank with wide legs will give you stability when you perform the Renegade Row.

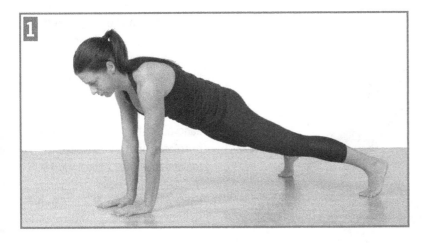

THE POSITION: Place your hands very close together on the floor and step your feet out behind you to form a straight line from head to heel. Widen your feet shoulder-width apart. Make sure that you can hold this plank for 30 seconds before moving on to Step 2.

continued on next page

continued from previous page

STEP 2: RENEGADE HOLD (ALTERNATING ONE-ARM PLANK)

This exercise makes sure that you can stabilize using one arm at a time.

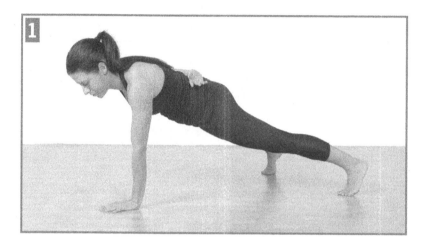

1 Continuing from high plank, bring one hand behind your back. Try not to twist or rotate your trunk. Focus on the arm that is keeping you up and stabilize yourself.

Alternate putting each hand behind your back.

STEP 3: 1-ARM PLANK HOLD

Time to add the bells. *Warning:* Be sure to use minimum 12kg (25lb) bells and a stable surface.

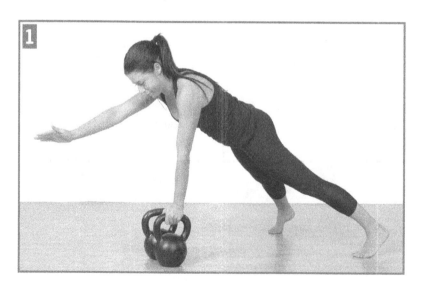

1 Assume a high plank with wide legs and place your hands on the handles of two upright kettlebells that are next to each other. Shift your body weight to make sure that the kettlebells are directly under your shoulders. Once you feel stable, raise one hand out in front of you. Try not to rotate your trunk during this movement—stay tight. Hold for 3–5 seconds. Focus on the arm holding you up, not the arm in the air.

Switch to the other hand.

Make sure you can perform the Renegade Row Prep exercises (page 87) before trying this.

STARTING POSITION: Assume a high plank with wide legs (Step 1) with your hands on the handles of two upright two kettlebells that are next to each other.

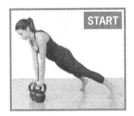

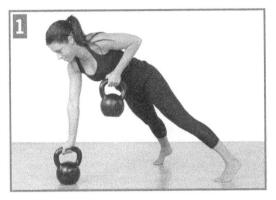

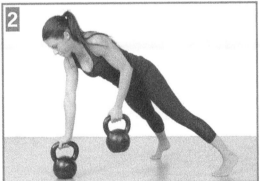

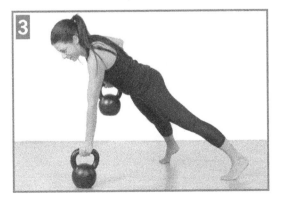

1 Stabilizing yourself on one arm, row the other arm up by bringing the bell to your rib cage. Be sure to keep your hips as level as possible.

2 Slowly lower the bell back down with control.

3 Focusing on the arm that's holding you up, shift to the other side and perform a row with your other arm.

TIPS

• *Use compression breaths (i.e., hissing or sissing noises) during Renegade Rows to brace your abdominals. These will give you abs of steel.*

STARTING POSITION: Take a wide stance with your right leg forward, foot pointing straight ahead, and left foot perpendicular; bend your right knee as if for a lunge. Place your left hand on the kettlebell on the floor to the inside of your front foot. Keeping your back flat, rest your right forearm gently on your thigh to stabilize.

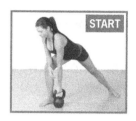

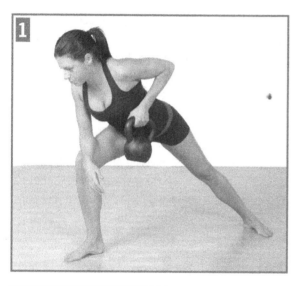

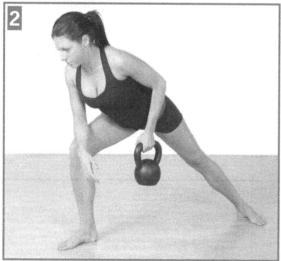

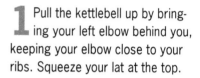

1 Pull the kettlebell up by bringing your left elbow behind you, keeping your elbow close to your ribs. Squeeze your lat at the top.

2 Slowly lower the kettlebell back down to starting position.

STARTING POSITION: Stand with your feet shoulder-width apart and hinge your hips behind you while keeping a flat back. Place your hand firmly against a flat, raised surface, and lock out your arm. The kettlebell should be on the floor beneath your shoulder. Balance your weight by placing your free hand on the handle without letting your shoulder drop.

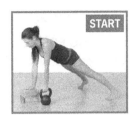

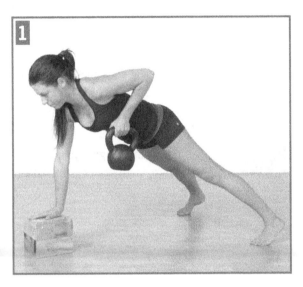

1 Exhale and pull the kettlebell off the ground by bringing your elbow back behind you.

2 Inhale and slowly lower the kettlebell back to the floor with control.

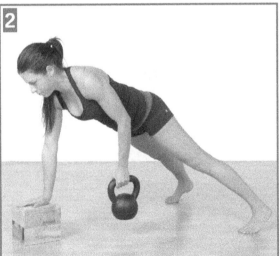

Warning: Don't do this exercise if you have a weak back.

STARTING POSITION: Stand with your feet shoulder-width apart and shift your hips back behind you. Place your hands on the two bells on the floor between your feet.

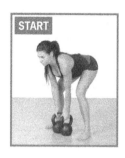

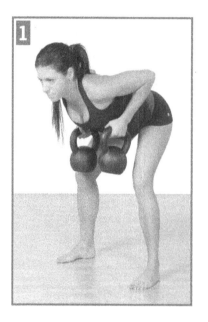

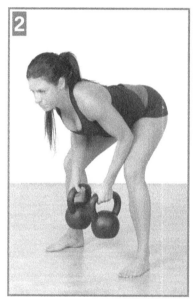

1 Keeping your back flat, exhale and pull both bells off the floor, driving your elbows back behind you.

2 Without changing your posture, lower the bells back to the floor.

STARTING POSITION: Stand with your feet shoulder-width apart and your hips shifted back behind you. The bell is on the floor between your feet. Keep your back flat throughout the exercise.

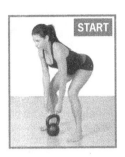

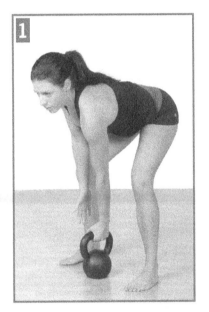

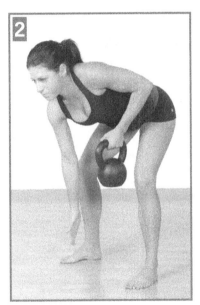

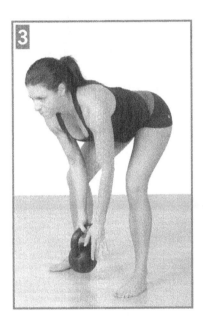

1–2 Reach for the bell with one arm and then drive your elbow up.

3 Lower the bell down to the floor with control and switch hands.

Arm-Sculpting & -Strengthening Drills

These next few exercises isolate the triceps, biceps, and even the lats. Although they're not required for a shredded look, isolating these muscles from time to time is an easy way to keep them strong.

TRICEPS EXTENSION

Use a lighter bell when you first start learning this exercise.

STARTING POSITION: Stand with your feet shoulder-width apart and hold the kettlebell by the ball with the handle between the index finger and thumb of both hands. Keeping your elbows straight, raise the kettlebell up over your head.

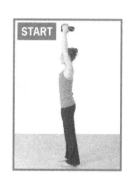

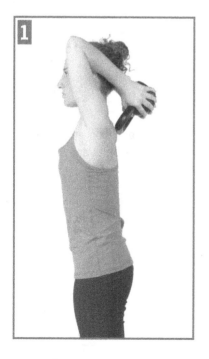

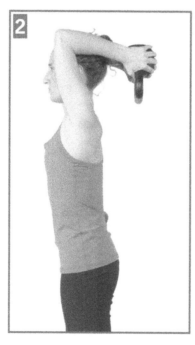

1 Keeping your elbows close together, lower the kettlebell behind your head.

2 Squeezing your glutes, bring the kettlebell back up over your head, straightening your elbows at the top.

STARTING POSITION: Stand with your feet shoulder-width apart and hold the kettlebell by the horns, keeping your arms straight.

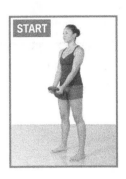

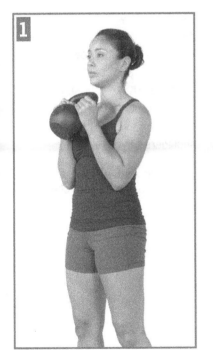

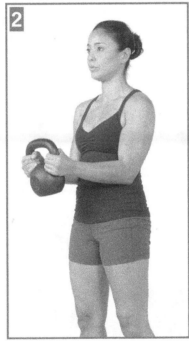

1 Keeping your elbows close to your sides, curl the kettlebell to your chest.

2 Slowly lower the kettlebell with control back down until your arms are fully extended.

This great exercise for strengthening your lats is a nice stretch as well.

STARTING POSITION: Lie on your back with your knees bent and feet flat on the ground. Hold the kettlebell by the ball with the handle between the thumb and index finger of both hands. Press the bell over your chest.

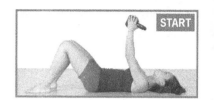

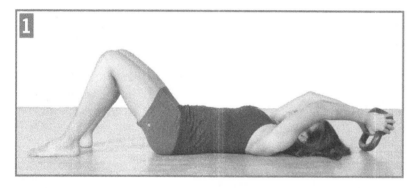

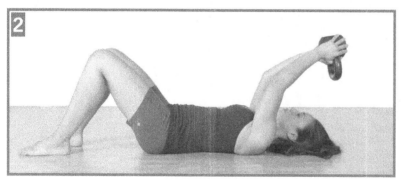

1 Keeping your arms straight except for a slight bend in your elbows, inhale and slowly lower the kettlebell toward the floor behind your head. Keep your shoulders and neck fully relaxed throughout the exercise—don't bring your shoulders to your ears.

2 Using your lats, pull the kettlebell back over your chest.

STARTING POSITION: Lie on your back, holding the kettlebell by the ball with the handle between the thumb and index finger of both hands. Bend your knees and raise your feet off the floor. Press the bell over your chest.

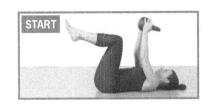

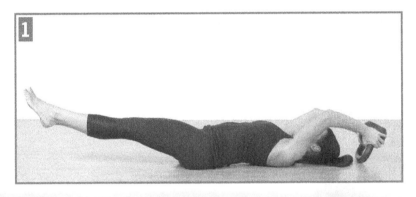

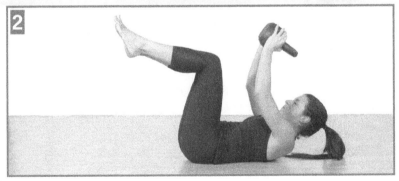

1 Keeping your arms straight except for a slight bend in your elbows, inhale and slowly lower the kettlebell toward the floor behind your head, extending your legs out slightly.

2 Pull the kettlebell back over your chest as you simultaneously bring your knees in toward your chest. Only lift your shoulder blades off the ground. Make sure the bell goes over your knees.

Arm-Sculpting & -Strengthening Drills | **97**

Core Exercises

There isn't a single kettlebell exercise in this book that doesn't work the core. Kettlebells will strengthen the core extremely quickly due to the explosive power, compound motions, and intensity involved in all the movements. Keep in mind that many people may have a very strong core but still have high body fat. If you want to see your strong abs, a combination of cleaning up your diet and smart training will strip the fat away, allowing you to see all of your hard work. These exercises really isolate the core, which will help you get those abs of steel.

JANDA SIT-UP

This is a very slow exercise that should be challenging. Keep the reps low and pay attention to the breathing. It's also a very effective abdominal strengthener.

STARTING POSITION: Lie on your back with your knees bent and feet flat on the ground. Place the kettlebell on the floor between the arches of your feet, then squeeze the kettlebell between your feet and place your hands across your chest.

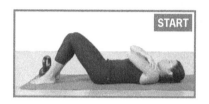

START

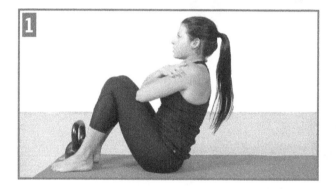

1 Using a slow compression breath (with a hissing sound), slowly sit up by bringing your chest up toward your knees.

2 Squeeze your glutes and slowly lower yourself to the ground.

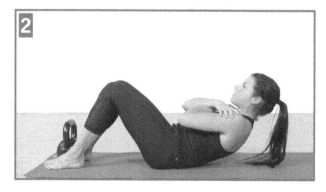

SIDE PLANK

When done correctly, this is great for strengthening the obliques, lats, and arms.

STARTING POSITION: Assume a high plank position.

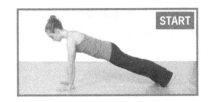

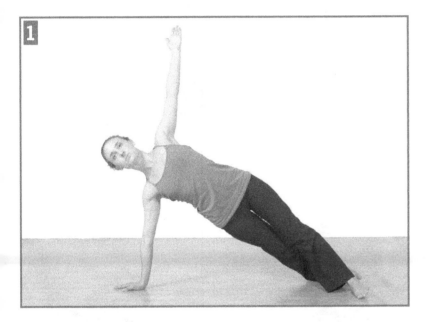

1 Raise your left arm off the ground and turn your whole body open to the left side. Your right hand will be flat on the ground and your feet will be staggered. Keep your hips high and your shoulder packed into your arm. Keeping your neck long, reach your free hand to the ceiling. Hold for 20–30 seconds.

Switch sides.

ALTERNATING VARIATION: To make this more challenging, shift to the side plank on one side and hold for 3 seconds. Rotate your body back into the high plank and hold for another 3 seconds. Open up to the other side and hold for 3 seconds. Continue switching and holding, working your way up to a minute.

KETTLEBELL VARIATION: This can also be done by balancing one hand on the kettlebell.

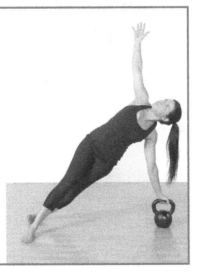

STARTING POSITION: Sit on the floor with your knees bent and heels off the ground, holding the kettlebell by the horns.

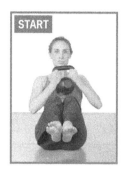
START

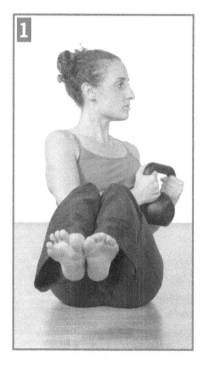

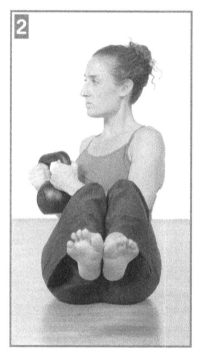

1 Gently rotate the kettlebell to the left side of your torso. Quick exhales on each rotation keep the core tight.

2 Gently rotate the kettlebell to the right side of your torso.

VARIATIONS: Place your feet on the ground if your lower back is weak. Lean back to make it more challenging.

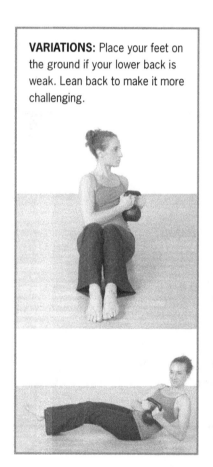

STARTING POSITION: Stand with your feet shoulder-width apart, holding a light kettlebell in the palm of one hand.

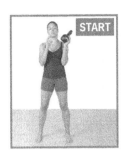

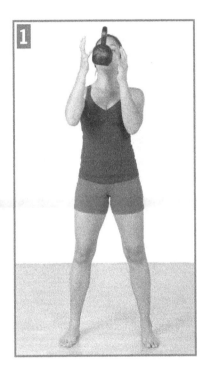

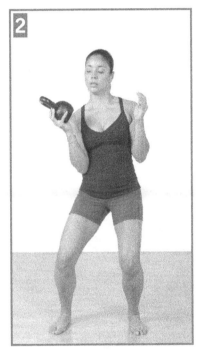

1–2 Toss the bell from one hand to the other quickly as if you're holding a hot potato, always keeping your elbows close to your body. Soften your knees with a slight dip when you toss it to make catching the bell easier.

Continue passing it back and forth, staying soft and relaxed as you pass, but keep your arms tight against your body.

FIGURE 8

The goal is to make a figure 8 between your legs.

STARTING POSITION: Stand with your feet shoulder-width apart and hold the bell in your left hand.

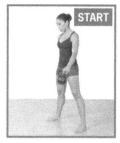

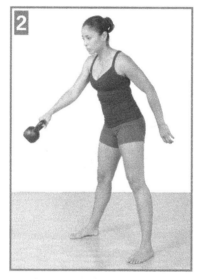

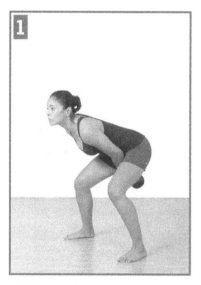

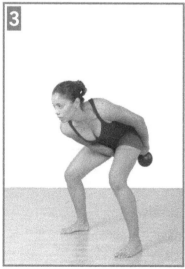

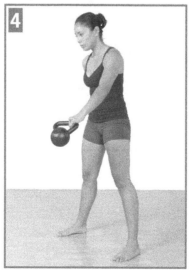

1 While hinging your hips behind you, pass the bell through your legs to your right hand.

2 Bring the bell around the outside of your right leg while snapping your hips forward and standing tall.

3–4 Pass it between your legs again, this time passing the bell to your left hand and bringing it around your left leg.

FIGURE 8 TO HOLD

This exercise adds a gentle swing.

STARTING POSITION: Stand with your feet shoulder-width apart and hold the bell in your right hand on the outside of your right leg.

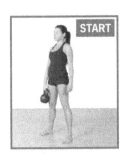

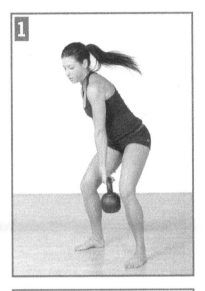

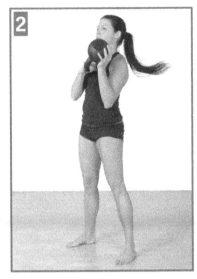

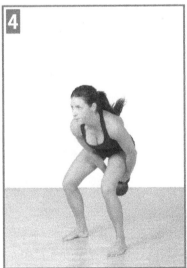

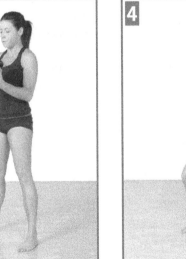

1 Hinge your hips back and gently hike the kettlebell back with your left hand. Reach behind your right leg and pass the bell to your right hand.

2 Thrust your hips forward and diagonally swing the bell up to your left shoulder, catching it with the palm of your hand. Don't let go.

3 Release the bell from the palm of your hand by gently pushing it away.

4 Weave it through your legs by passing it behind you to the other hand.

Continue weaving the kettlebell around your legs to create a figure 8.

Squats

Squats, hands down, are one of the best leg exercises you can possibly do. They not only help you develop strong legs, they increase flexibility and mobility in your hip flexors and knees. Squats strengthen the core using abdominal pressurization with added weight.

SQUAT

This is the basic movement for all kettlebell squats. Make sure you can do the squat without any weight before loading up.

STARTING POSITION: Stand with your feet anywhere from hip- to shoulder-width apart. Plant your heels and toes firmly on the ground; you may have a slight toe turnout.

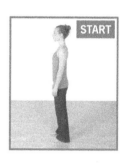

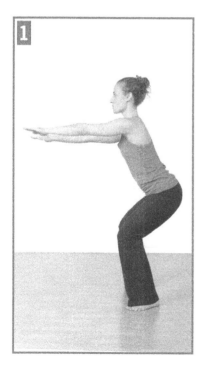

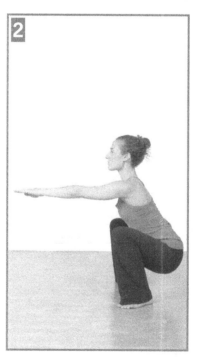

1–2 Hinging your hips back behind you, inhale and bend your knees, slowly lowering yourself past your knees; you may extend both arms forward for balance. Make sure that your toes track your knees. Allow your knees to open up to get lower in your squat. Keep your head forward and your spine as straight as possible.

3 At the bottom of the squat, brace your core with a compression breath before exhaling to stand back up. Immediately squeeze your glutes when you reach the standing position.

TIPS

• *Keep your knees pushed open on the way up and down. DO NOT allow your knees to collapse inward with any squats. This may lead to knee injury.*

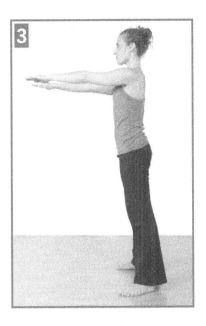

GOBLET SQUAT VARIATION:
Perform the squat while holding the kettlebell by the horns.

FRONT SQUAT VARIATION:
Perform the squat with a kettlebell in rack position. Keep the bell firmly in rack position throughout the movement—DO NOT let the bell get away from you.

DOUBLE FRONT SQUAT VARIATION: Perform the squat with two kettlebells in the rack position. The heavier the load, the more important the breathing. Sniff through your nose, descend to the bottom position, and grunt or hiss back up to standing.

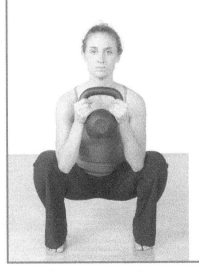

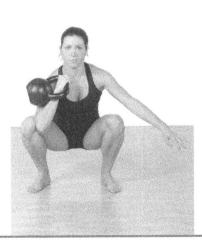

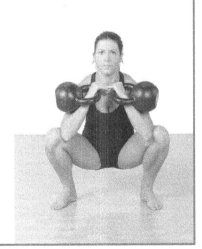

For the purposes of this book, we'll do the less-advanced version of the Overhead Squat. The upper portion of the descent will feel similar to the windmill. When first learning this exercise, start with a light kettlebell or no weight at all.

STARTING POSITION: Stand with your feet hip-width apart and a bell in one hand locked out over your head. Look straight ahead.

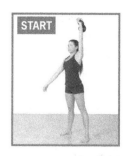

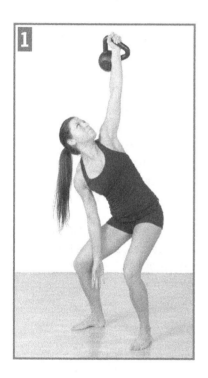

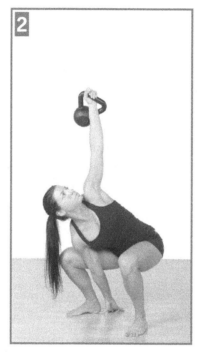

1–2 Turn your head to watch the bell while slowly lowering yourself down into a squat. Your torso will turn slightly as you descend. Reach your free hand through your legs and back toward the floor to keep your knees from collapsing inward. Drive yourself back up to starting position, squeezing your glutes at the top. You should be facing forward at the very top. Make sure to work both sides.

SINGLE-LEG SQUAT ON BENCH

This more-advanced version of the squat builds amazing strength and control in your legs. Start with a high bench and gradually work your way down to a lower bench as you become stronger and gain more control with this exercise. If you have limited ankle flexibility, holding onto a weight should be helpful for balance.

STARTING POSITION: Stand in front of a bench or chair and hold a small kettlebell by the horns close to your chest. Raise one foot off the floor, keeping the leg straight.

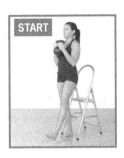

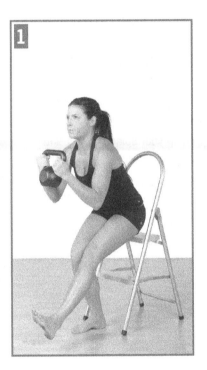

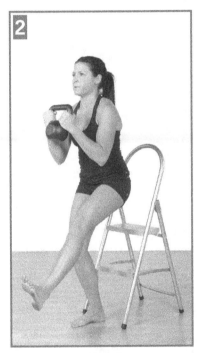

1 Shift your hips back behind you and slowly pull yourself down to the bench. Gently tap the bench with your rear end. Do not rest on the bench.

2 Push through your entire foot to grind yourself back up. Your glutes and quads should be tight at the top.

When you can perform 5 great reps per side, try doing a single-leg squat on a step.

DECK SQUAT

This fun variation of the squat will get your heart pumping. Make sure that you've mastered the Bodyweight Squat (page 132) before adding this squat to your arsenal. You'll want a mat or softer surface to protect your spine. I've done it on concrete and it's not very pleasurable.

STARTING POSITION: Take a comfortable stance with your feet anywhere from hip- to shoulder-width apart. Plant your heels and toes firmly on the ground. Hold a kettlebell by the horns for counterbalance.

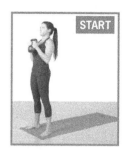

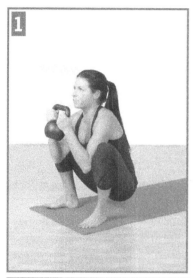

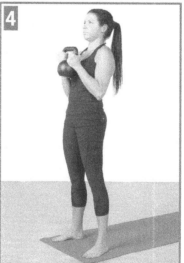

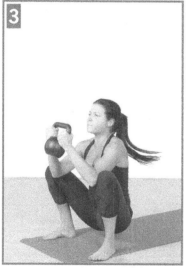

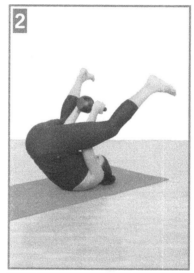

1 Hinging your hips back, slowly lower yourself down toward the floor. All the squat rules still apply!

2 Inhale and roll back onto the mat, keeping the bell close to your chest. DO NOT let the bell roll back over your head!

3 Rapidly exhaling, roll forward into the bottom of the squat. Keep your spine straight and aligned with the bell in front of you.

4 Stand up and squeeze your glutes.

Lunges

Lunges are a phenomenal exercise that not only work balance and stability, but help strengthen and sculpt your legs and glutes. Your core works as well to help stabilize.

STATIONARY LUNGE

If you're new to lunges, I recommend beginning your journey here. Feel free to start by holding on to a bench or wall for balance. Don't start adding weight until you have this movement pattern down perfectly without needing to hold on to anything.

STARTING POSITION: Step one foot forward and one foot back behind you in a split stance. Your front foot should be planted firmly on the floor while your back heel is off the ground.

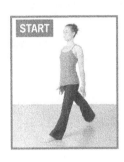

START

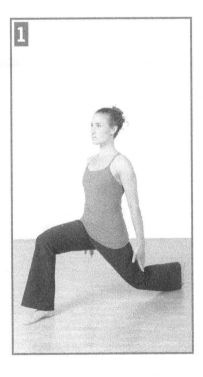

1

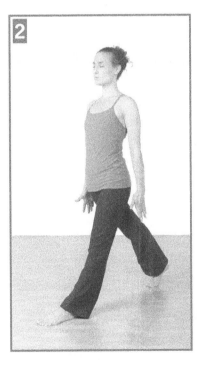

2

1 Bend both knees to lower your body down toward the floor until the back knee gently touches or gets close to the ground. Keep your front knee tracked along your front foot. DO NOT let your knee collapse inward.

2 Push through your front heel and back leg to return to the starting position. Squeeze your rear-leg glute at the top.

Switch legs.

TIPS

- *Be sure not to fold from your hips during the movement. Your spine should be perfectly straight.*

- *DO NOT lift your front heel.*

Once you feel proficient with the Stationary Lunge (page 109), you can add weight. Here we start with one bell to make it more challenging than the bodyweight version.

STARTING POSITION: Assume a split stance and hold one bell by the horns close to your chest. Keep your spine erect throughout the exercise.

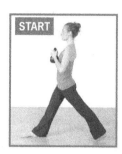

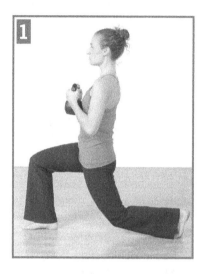

1 Lower your body into a stationary lunge. Make sure the bell doesn't cause you to fold over. Keep the bell by your chest for the entire duration of the rep.

Switch legs to work both sides evenly.

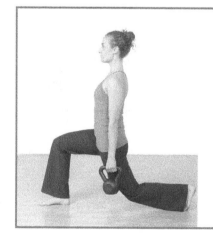

DOUBLE-BELL VARIATION: If you're feeling very strong with your stationary lunges, double kettlebells of the same size will really develop leg strength. Start with the bells on either side of your stance, lower down, and pick up the bells. Allow the bells to pull your shoulders slightly back and down. Keep the bells in your hands for the entire duration of the rep.

STARTING POSITION: Stand with your feet hip-width apart and the kettle-bell in your right hand in the rack position.

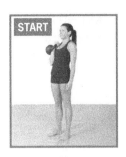

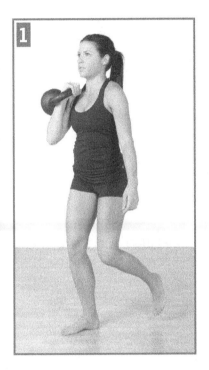

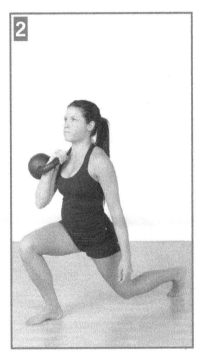

DOUBLE-BELL VARIATION: This can also be done with two bells in the rack position.

OVERHEAD VARIATION: Lock out one bell overhead and perform the lunge.

1–2 Step your left leg behind you and lower your left knee down toward the ground, keeping your torso upright.

Drive through your right heel and step your legs back together.

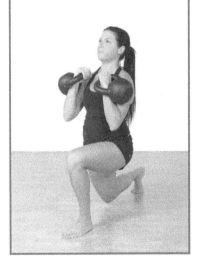

STARTING POSITION: Stand with your feet hip-width apart and hold a kettlebell by the horns in both hands.

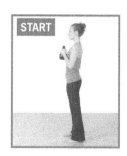

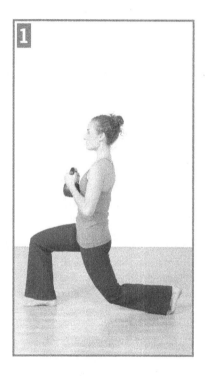

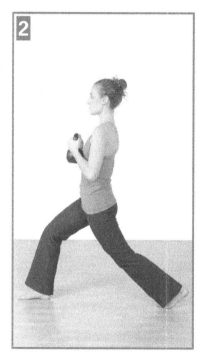

1 Step forward into a lunge with your right foot and firmly plant your front heel into the ground.

2 Push off through your front heel to step back to the starting position.

Switch sides.

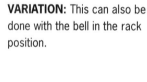

VARIATION: This can also be done with the bell in the rack position.

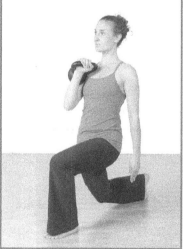

STARTING POSITION: Stand with your feet hip-width apart and hold a bell in your left hand, letting it hang in front of your left leg.

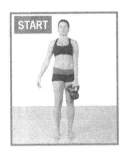

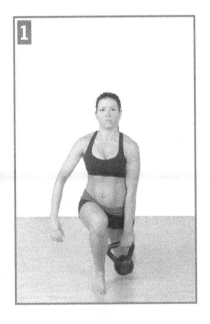

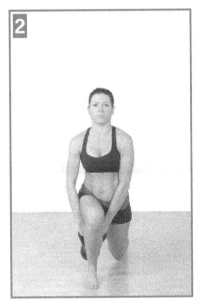

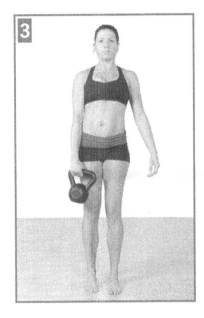

1 Step backward into a lunge with your left leg. Always lunge back on the side that has the kettlebell.

2 Pass the bell through your legs to your right hand.

3 With the bell in your right hand, step your left leg forward to the starting position.

Now lunge backward with your right leg and pass the bell to your left hand.

KICKSTAND LUNGE

This is a favorite exercise of mine because it breaks a lot of rules concerning the traditional lunge. The traditional lunges covered earlier in this section are all about keeping your spine aligned and focusing on your glutes, hamstrings, and quads in a balanced way. This lunge focuses mostly on the quadriceps because of the length of the stance.

STARTING POSITION: Stand with one foot in front of you and your back foot about half a foot behind you. Your back leg will only be used as your kickstand, therefore most of the pressure will be on your front leg.

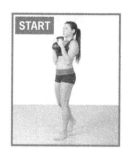

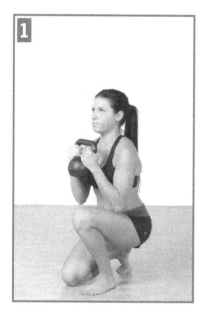

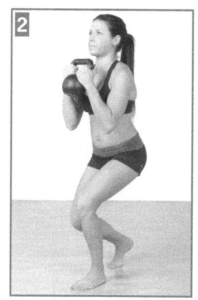

1 From a stationary position, lower yourself until your back knee is gently touching the ground. Because of the close stance, your hips will fold as you lower down.

2 Actively push through your front heel and stand upright.

MODIFICATION: If this is too challenging with the bell, you can practice without any weight.

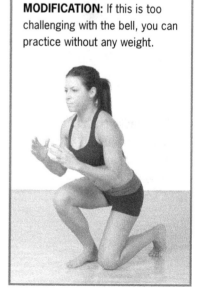

High Pull

The high pull is a cross between a 1-Arm Swing (page 50) and a Kettlebell Snatch (page 123). Many kettlebell instructors will introduce the high pull to teach the snatch. This is definitely an intermediate-level exercise. Make sure you have your 1-arm swing down before learning the high pull. The high pull works the glutes, core, lats, and shoulders, and has the same conditioning properties as the swing. It's also very fun once you master it as an exercise on its own.

HIGH PULL

STARTING POSITION: Set yourself up for the 1-Arm Swing (page 50).

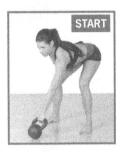

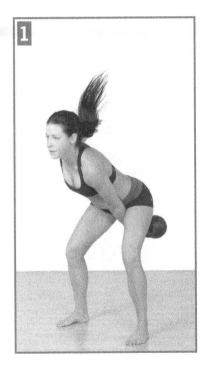

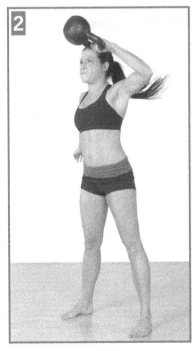

1 Hike the bell behind you.

2 Swing the bell forward and snap your hips while sharply pulling your elbow back at the top of the swing. The bell should be parallel to the floor, not drooping down. Think about elbowing someone next to you with power. Do not pause at the top because the bell will just fall.

continued on next page

continued from previous page

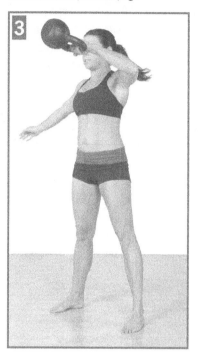

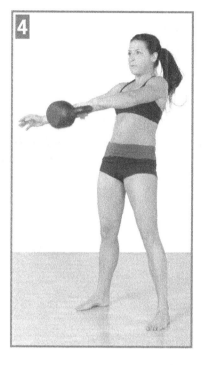

3–5 Now QUICKLY and immediately push/punch the bell back between your legs. Don't push it too far away from your body because you'll lose control of the bell.

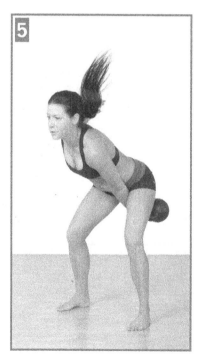

DOUBLE-BELL VARIATION: The High Pull can also be performed with two bells. This is one of my favorite exercises.

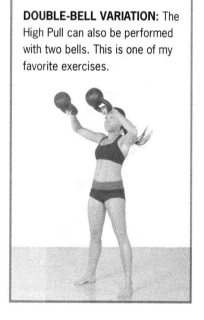

Turkish Get-Ups

This outstanding, full-body exercise will force your body to learn how to work together as one synchronized unit. Targeting the shoulders (deltoids), lats, abdominals (including transverse abdominis, rectus abdominis, and obliques), legs, glutes, and forearms, it's great for improving flexibility, shoulder stability, and core strength. Its benefits carry over into everyday life, and it'll also make all other overhead drills seem much easier.

When you first start learning this exercise, don't use a kettlebell. As you learn the proper movements and become more familiar with them, add a light bell. Don't be intimidated by all the steps. Patiently learn them and they'll all come together more easily than you think. Practice, practice, practice!

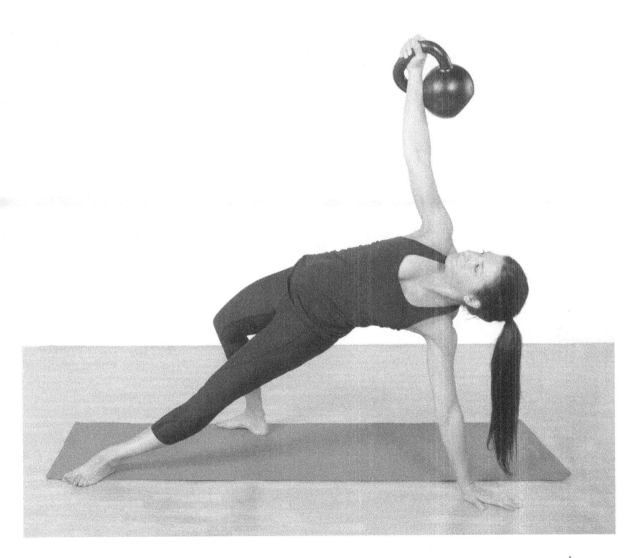

STARTING POSITION: Lie on your back with your legs straight and together and the kettlebell on your right side. Use the Floor Side Roll Pick-Up Method (1 Bell) (page 81) to get one bell into position in your right hand. Keeping your eye on the kettlebell and keeping your right arm and wrist straight, press the bell toward the ceiling.

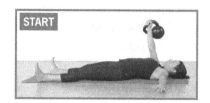

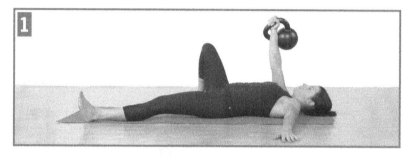

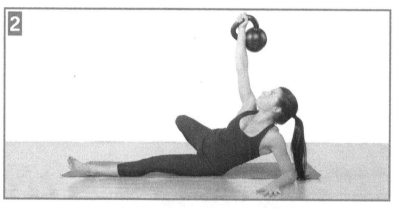

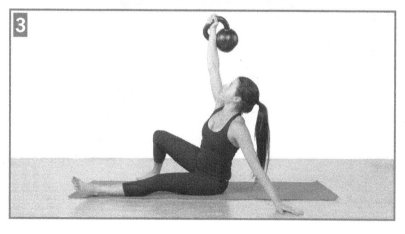

1 Step your right foot out to about a 45-degree angle. Your left hand will be on the floor away from your body.

2–3 Roll up and over onto your elbow then onto your left hand. Sit up while keeping the bell vertical.

TIPS

• Exhale with every step.

• Lead with your sternum. Don't allow your shoulders to cave in.

• Keep both shoulders pulled down and away from your ears.

The full Turkish Get-Up continues from the Get-Up Sit-Up (page 118).

STARTING POSITION: Perform the Get-Up Sit-Up.

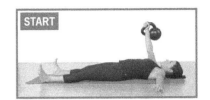

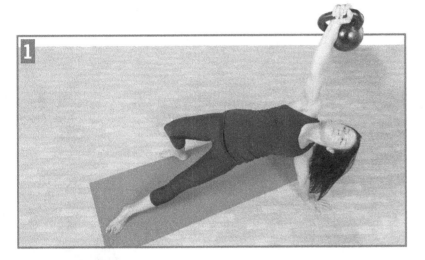

1 Lift your left hip up to create space in order to bring your left leg back behind you. (If you have great mobility, feel free to do the high bridge for this step).

2 Sweep your left leg back behind you, bringing your left knee close to being aligned with your left hand.

3 Release your left hand from the ground while keeping your right shoulder packed and down.

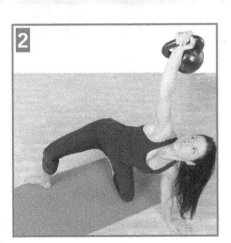

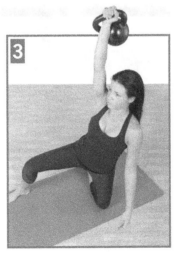

continued on next page

continued from previous page

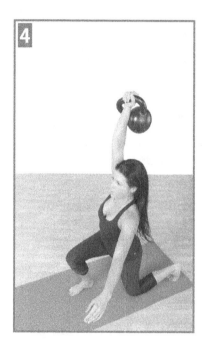

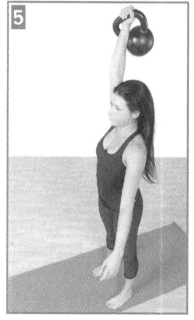

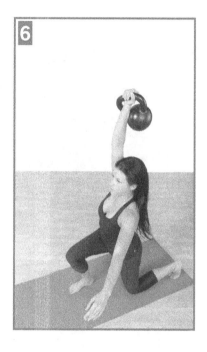

4 Windshield-wiper your left foot and adjust your front leg so that you're in a kneeling lunge position. Your back toes should be curled under. You can now look straight ahead rather than looking up at the kettlebell. The bell needs to be in a secure overhead lockout position.

5 Push through your front heel and back leg to stand up.

6 To get down, reverse the process by stepping back and down with the opposite (left) leg that the bell is on.

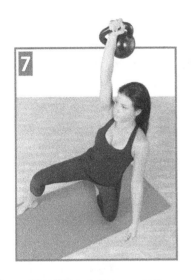

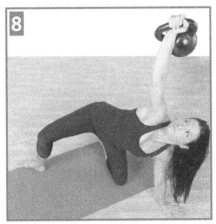

7 Windshield-wiper your left foot.

8 Shift your hips to the right in a windmill fashion as you reach for the ground with your left palm. This is when you should start looking at the bell again in your right hand.

9 Sweep your left leg back through and place your hip down.

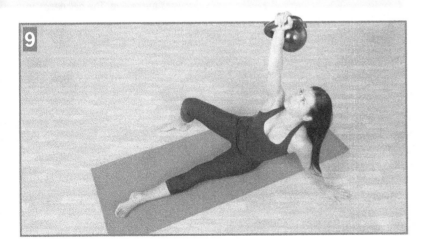

continued on next page

continued from previous page

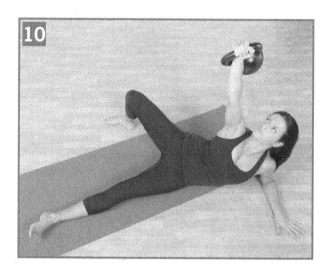

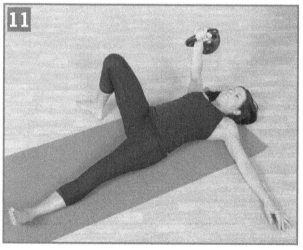

10 Slowly come back down with your elbow touching the ground first and then your back.

11 Safely roll the bell to the right to return it to the ground, unless you plan on performing another rep on that same side.

TIPS

• Keep your shoulder in its socket with your arm straight and the bell always toward the ceiling. The bell needs to be vertical at all times.

• Always keep an eye on the bell when getting up and down (except for steps 3–7, as mentioned above).

Snatch

According to Pavel Tsatsouline, the snatch is the tsar of all kettlebell lifts. It's the exercise used for testing, instead of push-ups, in the Russian Armed Forces. This exercise is catching on very quickly within elite U.S. military and governmental units, such as the U.S. Secret Service Counter Assault team. They're required to test with a 24kg (53lb) kettlebell for 10 minutes.

I've included this advanced exercise in my book because of how effective and fun it can be when done correctly. This challenging exercise builds very strong backs, hips, shoulders, and hands, as well as quickly increases your cardio power. Like the kettlebell swing, the snatch has a wonderful carryover effect to many different activities (e.g., running, jumping, fighting, board sports). I highly recommend that you spend ample time practicing this exercise. If you have sensitive forearms and wrists, you may want to look into purchasing wrist bands for the practice part.

SNATCH

STARTING POSITION: As with the 1-Arm Swing (page 50), stand with your feet between hip- and shoulder-width apart and the bell on the floor about 12 inches in front of you. Hinge your hips back behind you, keeping a slight bend in your knees. Keeping your back flat, grab the bell's handle with one arm.

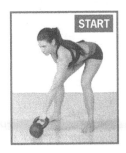

START

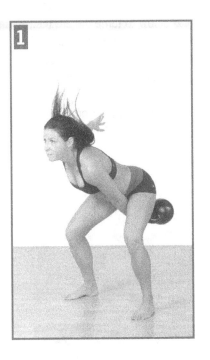

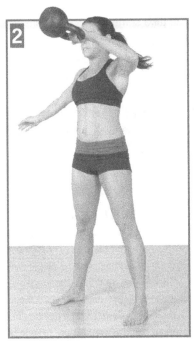

1 Driving your hips back, hike the kettlebell behind you.

2 Snap your hips forward to bring the bell up and then pull the bell back with a slight bend in your elbow. This is the pull portion of the snatch.

continued on next page

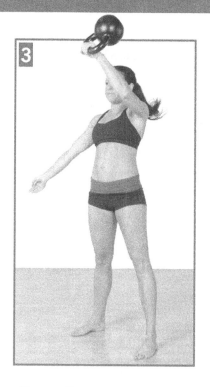

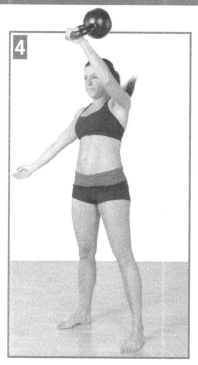

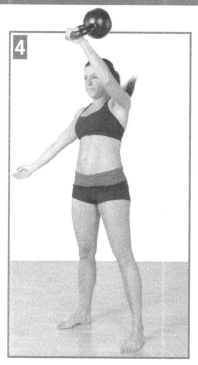

3–4 Quickly punch through the kettlebell with a relaxed grip, allowing the kettlebell to roll over your hand; in one uninterrupted motion your arm should be completely overhead in the lockout position. You'll need to loosen your grip on the handle in order for it to rotate easily in your hand. The bell should end up resting softly on your forearm without banging (this can take some practice). Think about beating the kettlebell to the punch! Make sure your elbow is completely locked out at the top of the snatch. Maintain this position for at least a second. You can open your hand at the top to allow blood flow back in.

5 Using a slight bend in your elbow to tame the arc (i.e., keep the bell close to your body), lower the kettlebell back between your legs. This will protect your shoulder, elbow, and back by not letting the bell yank on them.

TIPS

• Don't swing the bell up with a straight arm so that it flips over and bangs up your wrist.

• DON'T allow the kettlebell to yank on your shoulder during the drop part of the snatch. Lower and hike the bell back with control.

DOUBLE-BELL VARIATION: To make this exercise even *more* challenging, use two kettlebells. Don't attempt the double snatch until you've completely mastered the single-arm version. After you've snatched two kettlebells up at the same time and locked them out overhead, pull them both down to rack position before hiking them back between your legs for another rep.

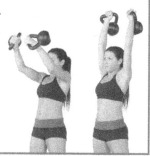

Warm-Up Exercises

Warming up should be a part of every workout that you do. Warming up properly can help prevent injury, make sure that the right muscles are fired up and activated, and allow you to ease into your workouts safely. Some of the warm-up drills will feel like easier versions of the actual workouts, but going through the motions should allow your body to loosen up and help create better blood flow for the entire workout. Think of these as pre-exercises for better performance. In the workout programs in Part 2, I've included days for just joint mobility and warm-up drills. Take 5–10 minutes out of your day to go through these exercises. You may also use these to cool down in addition to the stretches that are included in the cool-down section (page 145).

MINI PLANK

This amazing, simple-looking exercise was taught to me by Elise Badone, Muscle Activation Technique Specialist. It's incredible for firing the core muscles correctly before engaging in any activity. You'll literally feel your trunk muscles activating. It's perfect and a must for anyone who has experienced abdominal surgery, a hysterectomy, childbirth (natural or via C-section), excessive sitting due to a desk job, and any type of core weakness.

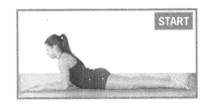

STARTING POSITION: Lie on your stomach on a mat with your elbows shoulder-width apart on the floor and your hands/forearms extended forward on the floor. Keep your chest off the floor.

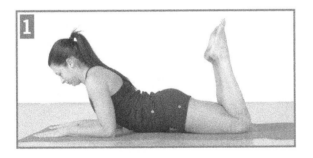

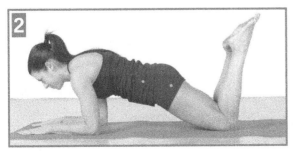

1 Keeping your knees on the mat, bring your heels toward your glutes.

2 Keeping your lower back straight, raise your hips to a plank position. Actively focus on bringing your pelvis to your rib cage to contract your abdominals. Hold for 6 seconds.

Lower your hips and then your legs. Repeat for 6 sets. Gradually work up to holding for 10 seconds each.

STARTING POSITION: Lie on your back with your feet flat on the ground, knees bent, and arms alongside your body.

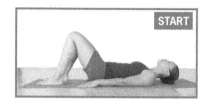

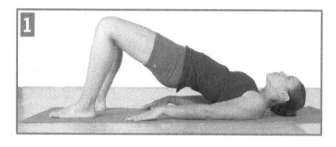

1 Pushing through your heels, lift your hips off the ground. Squeeze your glutes at the top.

2 Slowly lower down.

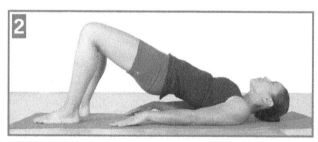

Only perform Single-Leg Bridges once you've mastered regular Floor Bridges (page 126).

STARTING POSITION: Lie on your back with your feet flat on the ground, knees bent, and arms alongside your body.

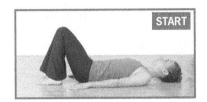
START

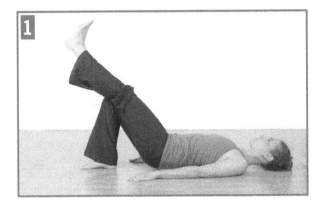

1 Keeping your knees beside each other, extend one leg out in front of you.

2 Push through the grounded heel and lift your hips.

3 Squeeze your glute and lower your hips.

Switch to the other side after you've done your reps.

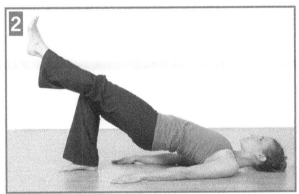

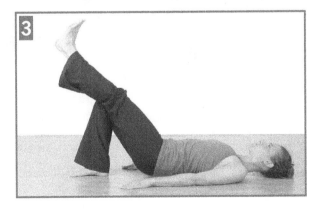

SQUATTING HIP OPENER

STARTING POSITION: Stand with your feet about hip-width apart.

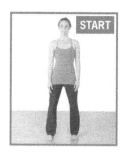

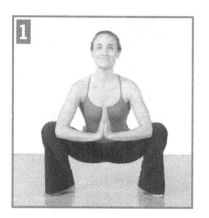

1 Reach your hips back behind you and squat down as low as you can comfortably go. Allow your knees to gently open up. Place your elbows against your inner thighs and gently "pry" your knees open.

HIP OPENER & GLUTE ACTIVATOR

This movement should be more of a circular motion.

STARTING POSITION: Assume a quadruped position, with your knees and hands on a mat and your back flat. Your hands will be directly underneath your shoulders and your hips will be stacked up with your knees.

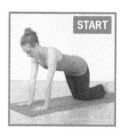

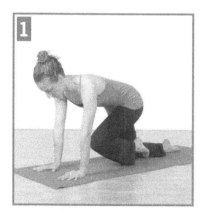

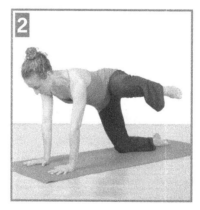

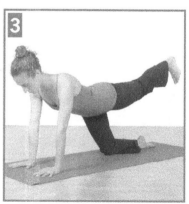

1 Bring one knee in toward your chest.

2 Laterally raise that knee out to the side to open up your hip.

3 Kick the leg out behind you.
Perform on each side.

ANKLE MOBILITY

Most people, especially women who wear heels or raised shoes on a regular basis, will have ankle mobility restrictions. Taking care of your tight Achilles tendons and ankle restrictions is key for a healthy body. When you lose ankle mobility, the domino effect of injuries down the line can be detrimental. Start dorsiflexing those ankles (i.e., bringing your toes closer to your shin) and take those high heels off! This particular exercise was taught to me by Functional Movement Specialist and Master RKC Brett Jones.

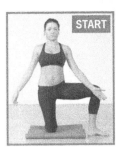

STARTING POSITION: Assume the open half-kneeling position, with your right knee on the floor while your left foot, hip-width apart, is aligned with your knee. Keep your pelvis straight.

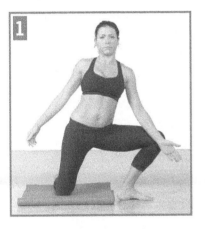

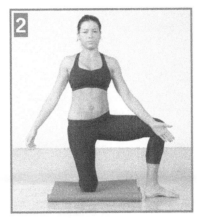

1 Keeping your left heel firmly planted on the ground, gently shift your body to the left so that your knee is over your toes. Hold for 1–2 seconds.

2 Return to starting position.

Perform on each side.

SHOULDER & THORACIC MOBILITY DRILL

STARTING POSITION: Lie on the ground in fetal position on your left side with your hips stacked atop each other and your arms extended in front of you along the floor. Neck and head support is recommended but not required.

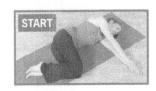

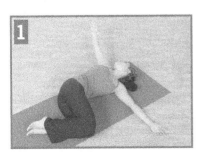

1 Bring your right arm away from your body and laterally toward the ground while turning your head to follow. Allow your rib cage to lift up and toward the open arm. You should feel a nice stretch in your shoulder and feel your thoracic spine open up.

STARTING POSITION: Standing with your legs shoulder-width apart, hold a light kettlebell by the horns with the bell up and handle down.

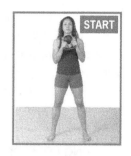

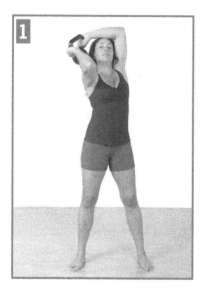

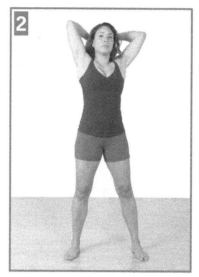

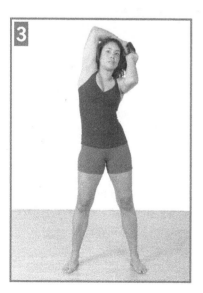

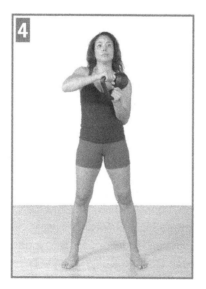

1-4 Starting with the upside-down bell at chest level, make a circle with the bell by rotating it all the way around your head. The bell will start to rotate and will be upright when it's directly behind your head. Gently keep your glutes tight in order to protect your lower back. You should feel your shoulders opening up and your neck and shoulders should be relaxed.

Do an even number of reps for each direction.

TIPS

• *Make sure the halo is fluid and your shoulders do not become your earrings. Squeeze those glutes.*

This shoulder opener will also require more core and glute activation than the Halo (page 130).

STARTING POSITION: Kneel with both knees on a padded surface and hold a light kettlebell by the horns with the bell up and handle down. Keep your hips stacked vertically over your knees and your glutes tight throughout this exercise.

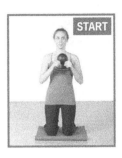

START

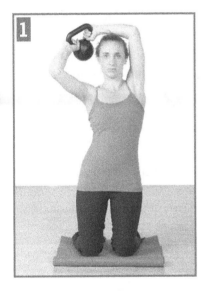

1

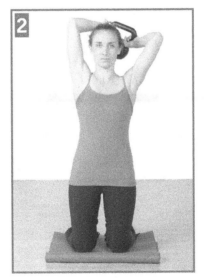

2

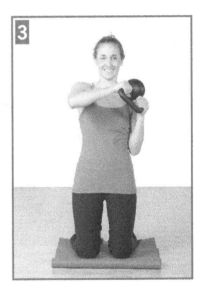

3

1–3 Starting with the bell at chest level, make a circle with the bell all the way around your head. The bell will start to rotate and will be upright when it's directly behind your head. You should feel your shoulders opening up. Gently keep your glutes tight to protect your lower back. Your neck and shoulders should be relaxed.

You'll want to do an even number of reps for each direction.

TIPS

• Make sure the halo is fluid and your shoulders do not become your earrings. Squeeze those glutes.

Doing 8 to 10 reps of these is a great way to warm up for your workout.

STARTING POSITION: Stand with your feet about hip-width apart.

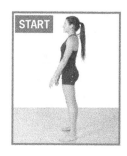

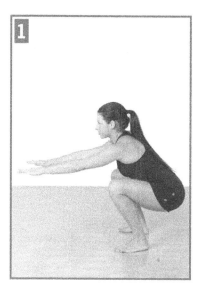

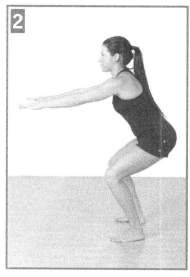

1 Reach your hips back behind you and down as low as you can comfortably go. Allow your knees to gently open up. You can have your hands directly out in front of you or keep your hands in close, using your elbows to "pry" your knees open.

2 As you return to standing, make sure your knees don't buckle inward. Actively push them open and squeeze your glutes at the top.

LATERAL LUNGE

STARTING POSITION: Stand with both feet together, pointing straight ahead. Extend both arms in front of you at shoulder height.

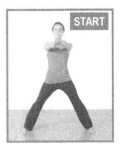

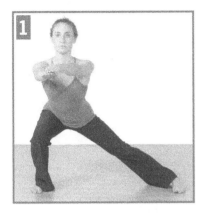

1 Take a big step out to the side and shift your hips back, bending the knee of the active "stepping" leg.

Step your foot back to the starting position. Perform on both sides.

FARMER'S WALK

Farmer's Walks are great at the beginning or end of any workout. They improve your core muscles, grip strength, and posture, and will get your entire body working.

STARTING POSITION: Stand as tall as you can while holding the kettlebell in one hand, letting it hang alongside your body with your shoulders pulled back and down.

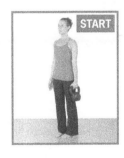

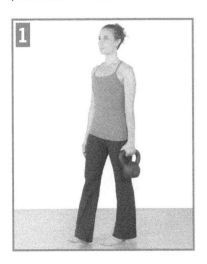

1 Using your core to stabilize, walk forward, making sure to stand tall. Don't let the kettlebell pull you over to one side.

DOUBLE-BELL VARIATION:
This can also be done with two kettlebells.

STARTING POSITION: Stand with your feet shoulder-width apart.

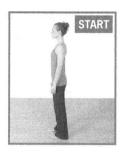

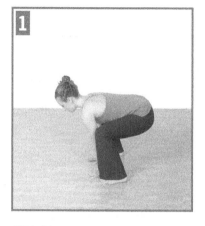

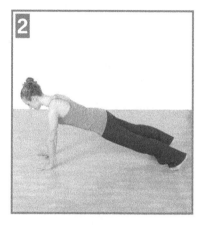

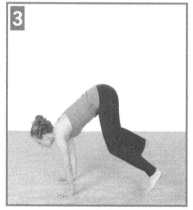

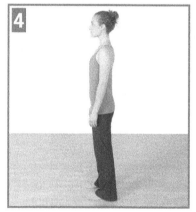

1 Squat down and place your hands flat on the ground in between your feet.

2 Jump your legs back behind you so that you're in a high plank position. Keep your core tight! Don't allow your trunk to sway to the floor as you jump your feet out behind you. Squeeze your glutes if you're not able to tighten your abs quick enough on the jump.

3 Jump your feet forward toward your hands.

4 Keeping a flat back, stand up.

BURPEE

The burpee is an advanced version of the Squat Thrust (page 134).

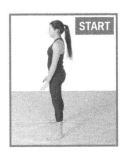

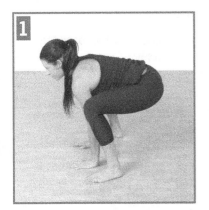

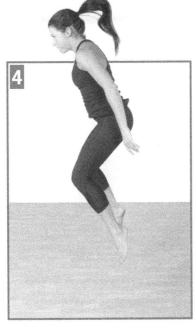

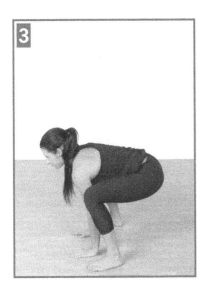

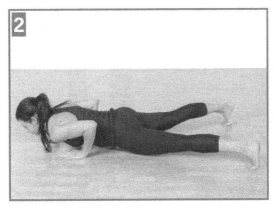

1 Squat down and place your hands flat on the ground in between your feet.

2 Jump your legs back behind you and perform a push-up.

3 Jump your feet forward toward your hands.

4 Explosively jump into the air, landing softly on both feet.

JUMPING JACKS

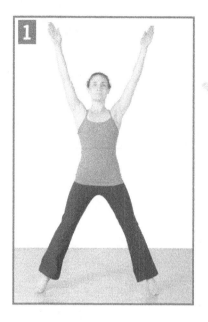 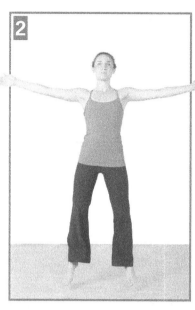

1 Stand tall, bend your knees and jump your feet wider than shoulder-width apart. At the same time, bring your hands up over your head. Stay light on your feet. To protect your back, keep your spine in neutral position. Only raise your hands as far as they can comfortably go.

2 Jump your feet back together and bring your arms down by your sides.

HIGH PLANK

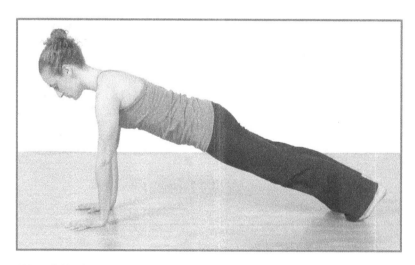

THE POSITION: Place your hands on the floor directly underneath your shoulders. Step your feet out behind you to form a straight line from head to heel. Keep your core stable and do not let your lower back sag.

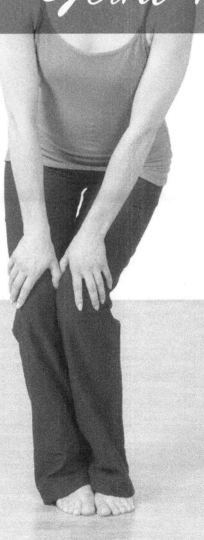

PART 4

Joint Mobility

Joint Mobility Exercises

Think about joint mobility exercises as an anti-aging pill for your joints. They can be done during warm-up, cooldown, or active recovery. By performing joint mobility exercises as frequently as possible, you allow the synovial fluid to keep your joints lubricated and mobile. Having strong muscles is one thing, but if you can't move through proper range of motion, your body will deteriorate very quickly. Do these exercises 10 minutes a day to keep your body as young as your mind. Generally, you should do each joint mobility movement for as many reps as your current age. For those who don't have that much time, something is better than nothing.

NECK MOBILITY: SIDE TO SIDE ROTATION

Don't force any of these movements.

STARTING POSITION: Stand with your feet hip-width apart and your hands relaxed by your sides.

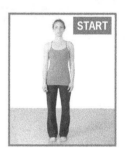

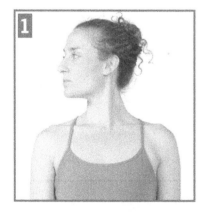

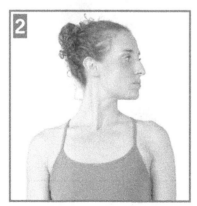

1 While keeping your body straight, turn your head to the right. Look as far back to the right as you can.

2 Repeat to the left, keeping your shoulders straight. Let your eyes follow your side-to-side neck rotations.

NECK MOBILITY: EAR TO SHOULDER

Don't force any of these movements.

STARTING POSITION: Stand with your feet hip-width apart and your hands relaxed by your sides.

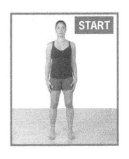

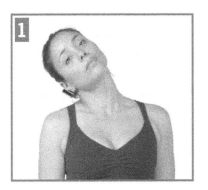

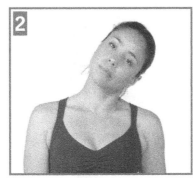

1 Keeping your shoulders down, gently bring your right ear down toward your right shoulder. You should feel a nice stretch in your neck and traps.

2 Gently return your head to the middle and bring your left ear down toward your left shoulder.

WRIST MOBILITY

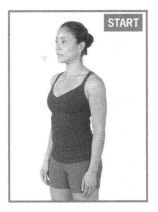

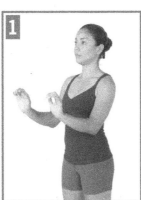

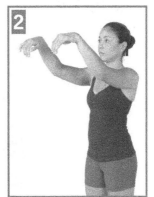

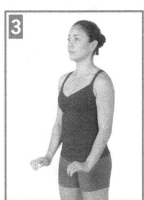

STARTING POSITION: Stand with your feet hip-width apart.

1 Bring both hands out in front of you, keeping your arms bent.

2-3 Move your arms up and down with loose wrists, like you're painting a fence.

STARTING POSITION: Stand with your feet hip-width apart.

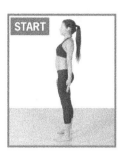

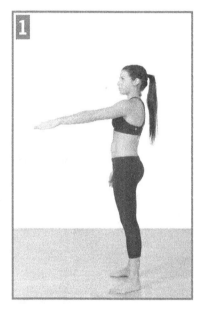

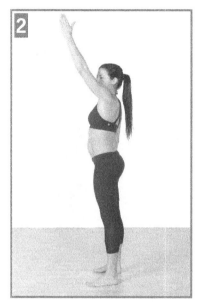

1 Straighten one arm out in front of you and gently lock out your elbow.

2–5 Paint a figure 8 in the air, allowing your shoulder to work through the different ranges of motion.

Switch arms and repeat.

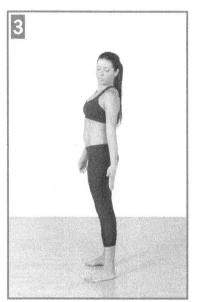

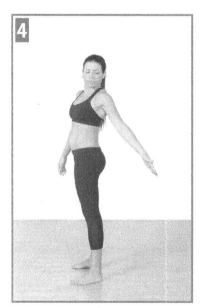

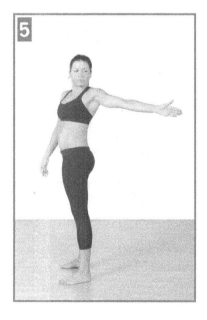

STARTING POSITION: Stand with your feet together. Bend your knees and place your hands above your knee caps.

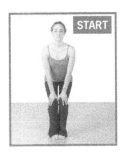

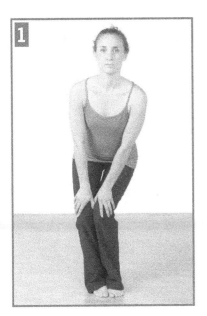

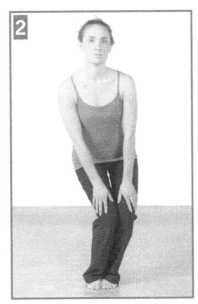

1–2 Move your knees around in a circular motion. You can gently straighten your knees each time. Don't hyper-extend them!

STARTING POSITION: Stand with your feet shoulder-width apart and your hands on your hips.

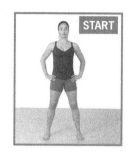

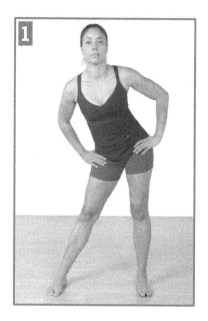

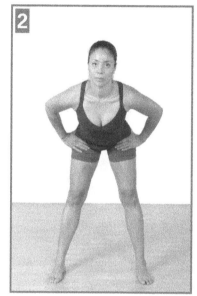

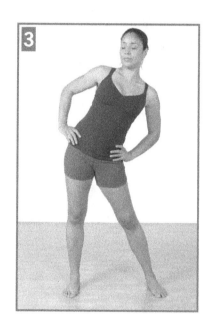

1–3 In a fluid motion, circle your hips forward, to the left, back, and then to the right.

Reverse direction.

STARTING POSITION: Stand with your feet hip-width apart and your hands on your hips.

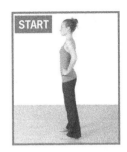

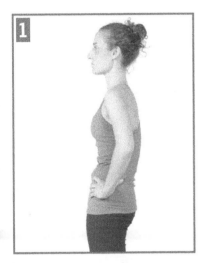

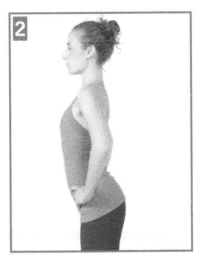

1 Tilt your pelvis forward.

2 Tilt your pelvis backward.

ANKLE CIRCLES

STARTING POSITION: Stand on one leg.

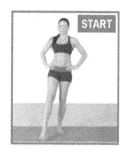

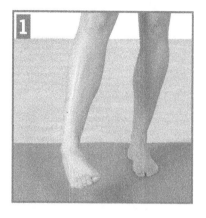

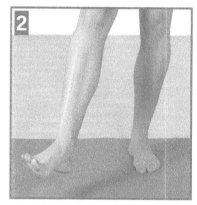

1–2 Rotate your other ankle in both directions.

Switch legs.

FINGER MOBILITY

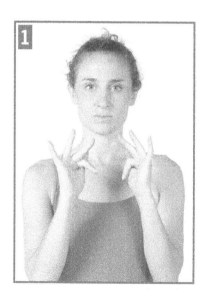

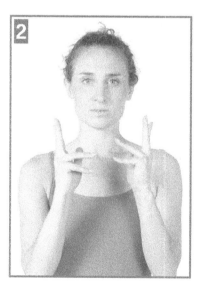

1–2 Stand with your feet hip-width apart. Starting with your hands wide open, press one finger down at a time until your hand is closed. Then reverse by pulling open one finger at a time.

Cool-Down Stretches

These stretches are best done after you've worked out and cooled down slightly but your body is still warm. The purpose of these stretches is to increase flexibility and range of motion. Choose the stretches that you feel your body needs and make sure to stretch both sides. Inhale deeply through your nose and breathe all your air out as you continue to further your stretch. Relaxed breathing is optimal during all of your stretches.

CHILD'S POSE AND LAT STRETCH

THE POSITION: On a mat, sit back on your heels with your knees hip-width apart. Reach out your hands to the floor in front of you while keeping your butt back on your heels. Spread your finger tips wide and allow your lats to feel this stretch.

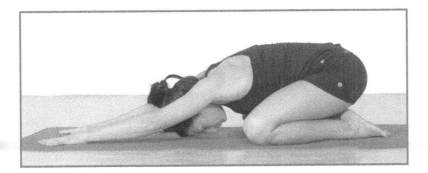

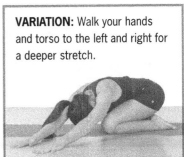

VARIATION: Walk your hands and torso to the left and right for a deeper stretch.

HAPPY BABY HAMSTRING STRETCH

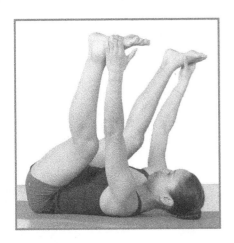

This is one of the best hamstring stretches that doesn't put any pressure on your lower back.

THE POSITION: Lie on your back and bring your knees toward your chest. Grab the outsides of your feet near the arches. Actively push your feet toward your hands, attempting to gently straighten out your legs. Unless you're very flexible, your knees will still be slightly bent. Hold for 15 seconds, back off, and then repeat 2–3 times.

This stretch is commonly used among Russian Kettlebell Challenge Certified and Functional Movement specialists. Not only does this give you more thoracic mobility, it stretches your shoulders, chest, and quadriceps as well. I originally learned this from Brett Jones. It has been nicknamed the "Bretzel."

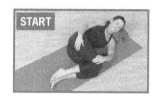

Caution: Don't force the rotation if you have any lower back issues.

STARTING POSITION: Lie on your left side with your head supported by a towel or block. Stack both hips atop each other while bringing your knees toward your chest.

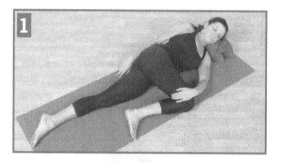

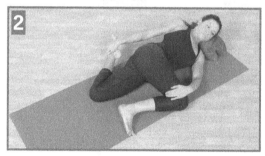

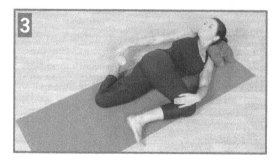

1 Keeping your right knee bent, straighten your left leg and place your left hand over your right knee.

2 Reach your right hand back for your left ankle. You should feel an opening in your chest.

3 Rotate your rib cage, not your lower back, toward your right shoulder and allow your head to follow your right hand, but keep your head rested on the towel. Make sure to take deep breaths and slowly allow your body to breathe more deeply into this stretch.

Switch sides.

OBLIQUE AND LAT STRETCH

STARTING POSITION: Stand with your feet hip-width apart and both hands over your head reaching as high as you can. Hold your left wrist with your right hand.

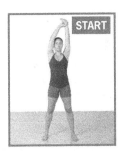

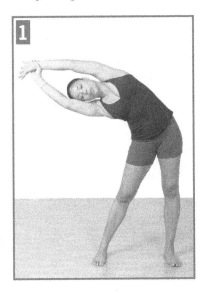

1 Gently pull up and over to the right side. Squeeze your glutes if you have a sensitive back. Hold for 15–20 seconds.

Switch sides. Repeat 2 times.

SQUATTING FIGURE 4 GLUTE STRETCH

THE POSITION: Stand and place your left ankle over your right knee cap. You may hold on to a wall for balance if needed. Hinge your hips back as if sitting in an imaginary chair. Find a point to concentrate on so that you can maintain your focus and balance during this pose. Hold for 15–20 seconds.

Switch legs.

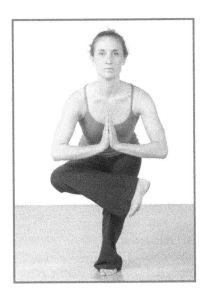

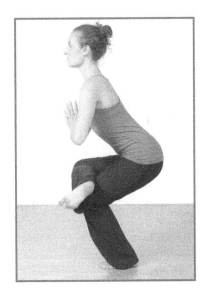

Index

Acknowledgments

I'd like to thank my husband Ben and my little girls Lyla and Chloe for being so supportive and understanding while I spent many hours away from them to write this book. Having their support and encouragement were a huge part of my ability to succeed. I'd like to also thank my parents, step-parents, and in-laws for being so encouraging throughout my kettlebell career. A big thank you to Dragon Door, all the RKCs, John Du Cane, Pavel, Brett Jones, and Mike Mahler for believing in me and being such great teachers. Thanks to my dedicated students in my kettlebell class, my loyal fans, and my followers who enjoy my no-nonsense approach to fitness. Last but not least, I'd like to thank the Ulysses Press team for choosing me to be their *Kettlebells for Women* writer and editor Lily Chou for being patient with me throughout the process.

About the Author

LAUREN BROOKS, the owner of On the Edge Fitness and BuggyBellz, is the creator of the highly acclaimed three-volume DVD series *The Ultimate Body Sculpt and Conditioning with Kettlebells*. She is also the creator of *Baby Bells*, the only pregnancy kettlebell DVD that exists as this book goes to press, as well as several other DVDs. The writer of many online and print fitness and nutrition articles, Lauren is also the creator of a new kettlebell iPad app. She emphasizes nutrition, lifestyle, exercise, and a positive mental attitude, and offers online nutrition and workout programs, as well as popular workshops worldwide. Lauren earned her B.S. in kinesiology with an emphasis in fitness, nutrition, and health from San Diego State University in 2002. She became kettlebell certified under Pavel Tsatsouline in 2005 and currently holds certifications as a Russian Kettlebell Instructor Level 1 and 2, RKC Team Leader, ACE Fitness Trainer, Clinical Nutritionist, Functional Movement Specialist, TRX, and Battling Ropes.

Lauren is married and the proud mother of two little girls. Drawing on her own experience and research, she has had the privilege of inspiring thousands of people from all walks of life and helping them achieve their fitness dreams. Lauren believes that if you truly love something and have a passion for it, make it happen even if it's a long road to get there. Life is way too short to wait for the perfect moment or the easy route. Live your life with no regrets!

For more information, visit her website www.OnTheEdgeFitness.com and blog (kbellqueen.blogspot.com). Lauren encourages people to e-mail her with success stories, feedback, and questions at lauren@socaltrainer.com.

CPSIA information can be obtained
at www.ICGtesting.com
Printed in the USA
FSHW020059280721
83439FS

9 781612 430270